Fit Kids **Revolution**

The Parent's Diet-Free Guide to Raising Healthy & Fit Children

Jon Gabriel & Patricia A. Ronald Riba, MD

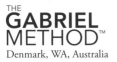

THE
GABRIEL
METHOD™
Denmark, WA, Australia

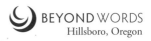

BEYOND WORDS
Hillsboro, Oregon

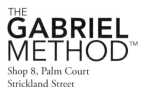

THE
GABRIEL
METHOD™

BEYOND WORDS

Shop 8, Palm Court
Strickland Street
Denmark WA, 6333
Australia
www.TheGabrielMethod.com

20827 N.W. Cornell Road, Suite 500
Hillsboro, Oregon 97124-9808
503-531-8700 / 503-531-8773 fax
www.beyondword.com

Copyright © 2014 by Jon Gabriel and Patricia A. Ronald Riba
Illustrations by Gabriela Menendez

The information contained in this book is intended to be educational and not for diagnosis, prescription, or treatment of any health disorder whatsoever. This information should not replace consultation with a competent healthcare professional. The content of this book is intended to be used as an adjunct to a rational and responsible healthcare program prescribed by a professional healthcare practitioner. The author and publisher are in no way liable for any misuse of the material.

Some names have been changed to protect the privacy of individuals.

First The Gabriel Method/Beyond Words trade paperback edition May 2014

The Gabriel Method logo is a registered trademark of The Gabriel Method Pty. Ltd.
Fit Club™, Fit Scouts™, and PC-Fit™ are registered trademarks of Dr. Riba's Health Club
Beyond Words Publishing is an imprint of Simon & Schuster, Inc., and the Beyond Words logo is a registered trademark of Beyond Words Publishing, Inc.

For more information about special discounts for bulk purchases, please contact Beyond Words Special Sales at 503-531-8700 or specialsales@beyondwords.com.

Manufactured in the United States of America

10 9 8 7 6 5 4 3 2 1

Library of Congress Control Number: 2014933174

ISBN 978-1-58270-520-0
ISBN 978-1-58270-527-9 (eBook)

The corporate mission of Beyond Words Publishing, Inc.: *Inspire to Integrity*

To the health, happiness, and prosperity of children around the world.

And to our own children, Ashley (Dr. Patricia's daughter) and
Inge (Jon's daughter), who are our best teachers, our most thoughtful critics,
our purest source of inspiration, and our greatest blessings.

CONTENTS

My Own Experience with Childhood Obesity by Jon Gabriel

"C'mon, Gabriel! Move it, you fat, lazy . . . !"

I heard this sort of abuse every day when I was younger. It was supposed to "motivate" me as I ran, mile after mile, day after day, in sweltering, summer heat. That was "fat camp," where loving, well-intentioned parents sent their overweight kids for summer vacation, putting them in the care of loving, well-intentioned, but highly misinformed, counselors.

The basic premise was simple: Isolate your overweight kids in a prison camp far from the temptations of and access to junk food. Severely restrict their calories and force them to exercise six hours a day for eight weeks. It was tough love, raised to an art form.

The result? Everyone lost weight, guaranteed. The only problem was that everyone would come back again the following year heavier than ever. We were limited to a bland, low-calorie diet that consisted mainly of things like thinly sliced Melba toast, reconstituted powdered eggs, grapefruit, and diet soda. Faced with this bland and nutritionally barren food, along with a punishing exercise regime, we'd look for a way out—any way out.

We would sneak out of camp, avoiding the imagined tracker dogs and searchlights, to go to the nearby truck stop and gorge on hamburgers, French fries, pies, and ice cream. We would eat so much that we could hardly walk back to camp. And when we couldn't get out, there was always the junk food black market.

Every summer, some daring kid would sneak out of camp and walk—or preferably hitchhike—five miles to a store to buy sweets. The enterprising, entrepreneurial camper would buy one box of forty Freihofer's chocolate chip cookies for two dollars and then sell the cookies for five dollars each.

We, the starving prisoners, were all so mad for those cookies that a simple sale would quickly degenerate into an auction, and often the bidding would go way beyond five dollars apiece. Sometimes money wasn't even enough. One time a kid, upset that my bid had won, ripped the cookies out of my hand and beat me up for them.

Looking back at the three years I went to fat camp, the weight gain yo-yo just kept getting worse. I got heavier each year, and I noticed that other kids got heavier each year too. This kind of pattern became a running joke. We'd lose 40 pounds in eight weeks and return 60 pounds heavier the next year, looking like someone had inflated us with some kind of air pressure pump. We all used to laugh about that. But it was no joke.

The weight loss never stuck. The second we got home we were like kids in a candy store again. The shackles were off, the food police were far away, and junk food was cheap and abundant. Some families would try to keep up the siege mentality in the endless war against calories by having locks on the refrigerators and pantries. My family had those locks too, but there was always, always a way around them, and I'd apply considerable ingenuity to figure it out. For example, the chain that went around the refrigerator had some play. The fridge could open just enough to stick a hand in and grab anything on the inside panel of the door. So my brother and I would plan ahead and always put the sweetest, most fattening foods within hand's reach. Being rebellious, sneaky, and above all *desperate* about food became a way of life. My brother and I once found some money on the street, and we went into a store and tried to figure out how to get the most calories for the money. Given our dedication to getting fat again, is it any wonder we succeeded, if you can call it that?

So why did we go to fat camp?

My father was overweight as a kid and suffered severe teasing and bullying growing up. More than anything, he wanted to prevent us from suffering the same fate. He knew the pain and suffering we were experiencing, bulging out of our school uniforms, being picked last for team sports, being spat on, and getting hit and taunted by smaller, faster children. He knew it all too well and would have moved heaven and earth to protect us from experiencing his pain. If being an overweight child is painful, and believe me it is, being the parent of an overweight child is twenty times more painful. All of their pain becomes our pain, magnified by feelings of shame, guilt, frustration, and desperation. And so out of love and with all the best intentions, my father became totally focused on solving our weight problem, and we became a "diet" family. My father was always researching the latest studies on weight loss strategies, and one after another, we tried them all.

First it was sunflower seeds. Sunflower seeds take some time to get into, so getting past the shell would force you to eat slowly, limiting the amount of food you could eat in any one time period. So when we'd go on an outing, we'd take bags of sunflower seeds with us and end up with bags and bags of sunflower shells.

Then it was "diet" candies. Only thirty-five calories each, these little artificially sweetened beauties tasted like laboratory floor dust wrapped in bubble gum. How the manufacturer managed to get them to taste so bad, I'll never know. But because they were purportedly "diet," we ate them like it was our last meal, day and night, for weeks. It turns out they weren't even diet at all. It was all a scam. They were actually sweetened with sugar.

Then Weight Watchers came up with a diet popsicle called the Chocolate Treat, which became the family's new diet food *du jour*. We ate Chocolate Treats all day. I remember offering one to my friend, and he laughed at me. When I questioned what was so funny, he said, "It sounds so doglike." It never occurred to me how strange it was to refer to food as a "treat," but he was right. He came from a family where food was only a very small part of the family experience. Food was always available anytime, and he ate whatever he wanted. He was a healthy, fit, active kid who probably never in his entire life thought to try to control what he ate; not even for a minute had he restricted the quantity or type of food he was eating. To him, food wasn't a treat, unless you were teaching a dog a new trick. I never realized it before, but growing up in my family, we had put food on some sort of pedestal, and yet, at the same time, food had been restricted, measured, and resisted, and every day was a fight, a battle between "good days" and "bad days."

Good days and bad days.

That's all we knew back then. That was our way of life. Most days were "good." We could fight our cravings, have the occasional "treat," and when we were good, we somehow managed to get through the day. But not every day.

It was usually on a Sunday night, every two weeks or so, when the whole thing would go out the window. We'd go to the local grocery store and buy two gallons of ice cream, plus chocolate cakes, chocolate sauce, and anything else we'd been hankering for, and we'd have a massive binge. Within two hours, we'd consume it all and end up feeling stuffed to the gills. Then Monday morning, we'd start the whole cycle again as if nothing had ever happened.

Let me be clear that my parents were always extremely caring and well intentioned. I always felt very loved and supported by them. I knew they had my best interests at heart. But unfortunately, they fell victim to the common myth of the time that weight loss is simply about calories in and calories out, and nothing more.

If there's one thing I know from firsthand experience, intense and in-depth research, and years of working with clients all over the world, it's that weight loss is not simply about calories in and calories out. You can force a child to lose weight in the short term by calorie restriction, but the feelings of chronic hunger and deprivation trigger emotional and biological changes that can cause a lifetime of weight issues. It's flawed logic because it doesn't factor into the equation the enormously complex intricacies of human biology. This flawed, oversimplified way of looking at the way that our bodies function is what Dr. Ron Rosedale, founder of the Carolina Center for Metabolic Medicine, calls "kindergarten medicine" and what I call the Flawed Diet Approach—an approach that still seems to underlie most weight loss methods.

What helped me conquer my weight problem in my early teens was a random conversation I had with my aunt when I was fourteen. I was making her a cup of coffee and asked her how many lumps of sugar she wanted. She said none. I couldn't believe you could drink coffee without sweetener. She said she used to drink coffee with lots of sugar and, in fact, she was addicted to sugar, but she did a visualization to break her addiction. She imagined sugar was ground glass, and when she ate it, it cut up her stomach. She said that after doing this visualization, she couldn't even *look* at a doughnut without becoming nauseous.

I had had a lot of experience with visualization. When I was ten, I suffered from severe migraine headaches. My headaches were excruciating and nothing, not even medicine, seemed to help. I used to lie in a dark room for hours and just endure the pain. This was nearly a daily occurrence for me. Out of desperation, my father tried a visualization technique to ease the pain. He was a dentist who used visualization for pain management as part of his practice. The technique was rather clever. He relaxed my body through suggestion and then told me to imagine that I was at the top of my favorite ski slope with a bucket of black sand on my shoulder. He told me the black sand was my headache. Then he guided me to imagine that I was skiing down this slope, and as I was skiing, the black sand was falling out of the bucket. Little by little the sand spilled out, and little by little my pain diminished. When we got to the bottom of the slope, the sand was gone and so was my headache. It was amazing.

I then learned how to practice this visualization myself with the same results. Eventually, I got so good at it I could get rid of a headache within minutes using visualization.

I knew the power of the mind from a very early age, and I knew the power of visualization. So when my aunt told me about her technique for killing her sugar cravings, I immediately tried it. And sure enough, it worked. From the day I practiced that visualization, I completely lost my taste for sugar. From the ages of fourteen to twenty-eight, I never once craved anything with sugar. Junk food was completely and instantaneously eradicated from my life.

During this time, I discovered competitive sports, and I started using visualization to help me train. I would imagine myself biking and running hard, lifting weights, getting into better shape, and being super successful at sports. This propelled me to become a competitive soccer player, ski racer, and eventually, a triathlete. And all my weight issues were solved once and for all. Or so I thought.

Unfortunately, in my thirties, I once again found myself on the weight loss and weight gain roller coaster. I managed to gain 220 pounds over an eleven-year period, calorie restricting and dieting the whole way up!

I started gaining weight in 1990 when I moved to New York City and began working on Wall Street. I was in a very high-stress job, working as a trading assistant on a bond desk. I was making $1,200 a month and my rent was $1,600 a month. To say that I was in a chronic state of fear and stress is an understatement. Stress can cause some people to gain weight, and I discovered I'm no exception to that rule. Stress can also cause junk food cravings, so my tastes for sugar and fattening foods came back too. I tried to resist my cravings, but no matter what I did, my body kept fighting me to gain more and more weight. My cravings were insatiable.

I'd go on a diet and lose 10 pounds through sheer force and willpower, but then I'd have a binge and gain the 10 pounds back and then some. Every diet I went on followed the same pattern. From low-fat to low-carb and everything in between, I would follow the diet to the letter, and I'd lose some weight. Then I'd fight cravings left, right, and center. The cravings would eventually lead to another massive binge, and I'd gain that 10 pounds back and put on another ten on top of that.

The dieting roller coaster continued. I'd lose 10 pounds, then gain 20 pounds, lose 10 pounds, then gain another twenty. I did this for eleven years, until cumulatively I had gained more than 220 pounds. I went from 185 pounds to 410 pounds, and even in the face of my repeated dismal failures, I'd continue to work hard to lose weight.

At one point, I had a weekly, face-to-face appointment with the late Dr. Atkins. Despite the fact that I had spent thousands of dollars on these appointments, one day, in sheer frustration at my failure to lose weight, he lost his temper with me. I was sitting in his office, and he looked at me and said, "What are you doing? You're killing yourself!"

I thought, *You are THE Dr. Atkins. You've sold twenty million copies of your book, and the best you can do is yell at me for being so fat? That's the best that you can do?*

It's not like I didn't have enough motivation to lose weight. I was getting up at seven in the morning and meeting with a fitness trainer before my meetings with Dr. Atkins. I had the motivation. I had the drive. I put in the effort. I just wasn't getting any results. My body was fighting me tooth and nail, and there was nothing I could do to stop it. Moreover, every other doctor I went to gave me that same look too, the same look that the fat camp counselors used to give me, the same look that all sorts of people were now giving me all the time—the look that said:

Oh, this guy doesn't care about himself. He's just weak and lazy.

However, I was far from weak and lazy. I met with doctors, naturopaths, homeopaths, acupuncturists, and anyone else I thought could help me. I could follow any diet to the letter, but I could only do it for so long. Eventually, the cravings would get to me, and I would binge. Then I'd start the whole vicious cycle again.

Atkins wasn't my only failure. I not only did the Atkins high-fat diet, but I also went to the Pritikin Institute and tried the low-fat diet. Each founder of every diet I tried had his own idea of what could work, and *nothing worked*. No doctor, no health professional, no acupuncturist, *nobody* understood the fact that my weight wasn't about me being weak or lazy or not caring about myself. I truly felt like my body was forcing me to gain weight.

My situation became critical in 2001 because by that time I'd reached over 400 pounds, and I'd become borderline type 2 diabetic.

Then I had my aha moment.

In August 2001, I was driving home from a movie and realized that I had no control over my body; I didn't understand why my body craved so much food or why my body gained weight so easily. The experts didn't know, and I needed answers. And then it hit me.

For some reason that I didn't understand, that nobody understood, my body just wanted to be fat and as long as it wanted to be fat—there was nothing I could do about it. This realization had a profound impact on me. I decided I was never going to diet again, and instead I would determine why my body was forcing me to gain weight and what I could *do* about it.

Even though I've attended the Wharton School of Business and have worked on Wall Street, I also have a solid biochemistry background from the University of Pennsylvania, with enough biochemistry, molecular biology, organic chemistry, physics, calculus, and anthropology coursework to attain a bachelor of science in biology with a minor in anthropology. I also completed a year of independent research into cholesterol synthesis with Dr. Jose Rabinowitz at the VA Medical Hospital in Philadelphia. I had even thought about going to medical school. All of this gave me a foundation for studying the latest research in biochemistry and obesity, as well as stress, a factor that I believed contributed to my weight gain.

I discovered a lot about the way our bodies really work and why so many of us put on unwanted fat. I learned how to properly nourish my body and deal with stress. I also started visualizing again. Visualization can be an incredibly effective tool for reducing stress, solving emotional issues, and achieving goals. Kids are great visualizers. Imagination comes so naturally to them, and I've had amazing success using visualization and guided imagery with overweight children.

I learned that obesity really wasn't the result of people being lazy or selfish or self-indulgent—this is especially true for children. There are real forces in our lives that trigger our bodies into putting on fat. I lived through it. I knew it was true. I was living in a body that was forcing me to gain weight. I knew there was more to the equation than just calories in and calories out. Moreover, I'd been on both sides of the tracks. From the ages of fourteen to twenty-eight, I had been effortlessly thin. Sure, I ate healthy and exercised, but it was all so easy. Eating healthy wasn't a chore. I didn't have any junk food cravings. Exercising was fun for me, and in fact, I didn't even need to exercise to be thin. Why then, all of a sudden, was it so impossible to lose weight? Why, despite the fact that I worked with the world's leading experts, did I just keep gaining and gaining?

Eventually, after I found the real, tangible answers to these questions and more, I lost more than 220 pounds of excess fat, and I've kept it off ever since. I've been the same weight since 2004, and maintaining this weight has been truly effortless. I eat what I want. I crave healthy foods, and I love leading a physically active life.

I've dedicated my life to spreading the message of what I've discovered, what worked for me, and what's now working for hundreds of thousands of men, women, and children all over the world, of all ages, in fourteen languages, and in sixty countries. And this is the message that I want to share with you, that we *do* have the ability to solve our children's weight issues once and for all if we look in the right direction and address the real issues.

First, you need to understand that there are real chemical reasons why your child is overweight. These reasons may have their roots in any combination of mental, emotional, or physical stress. These stresses cause our bodies to act like human fat storage machines. They activate a primal survival mechanism in our bodies I call the FAT programs, or the FAT switch. FAT stands for *Famine And Temperature*, which we'll get into in much greater detail in the coming pages. Simply put, turning off the FAT switch is the key. If you do that for yourself or your child, weight loss becomes easy and automatic. Your body actually helps you lose weight. It's not fighting you anymore. You become a naturally fit person, craving healthier foods and healthier portions and becoming naturally active.

I've now lived at both extremes of the obesity spectrum, and I can tell you, without a shadow of a doubt, that when you turn off your FAT switch, the struggle is over. The only struggle becomes understanding what's activating this FAT switch for you or your child, and then the rest is easy. And that's exactly what this book is about. This book is designed to help you understand your child's body and why it functions the way it does, so you can truly understand what your child is going through and give him or her strategies that address the root cause of the problem, eliminating it once and for all. This is not simply another approach that has you trying to force your kid to eat less, setting him or her up for yet another repeated failure. This book is about real causes and real solutions and empowering you and your child to help transform your child's body and life.

How I Became a Childhood Obesity Expert by Dr. Patricia Ronald Riba, MD

I have always been a fan of the underdog.

I find the plight of overweight children and their families to be extremely heartbreaking and challenging. The stories of children being bullied, teased, and shamed have touched and inspired me deeply. With the support of my mentor, Dr. Gwyn Parry, the Children and Families Commission of Orange County, and my amazing team, I have been able to live out my dream everyday by doing what I am passionate about.

For years, there have been no good answers to the question of childhood obesity, even though it has been on people's radars. Many well-intentioned people have forced themselves and their children to adopt unproven adult dieting concepts, like portion control. Because my team and I are in the thick of it—seeing the toughest cases in our county—I have seen firsthand that this approach is doing more harm than good. Over a decade ago, I was involved in Orange County's Childhood Overweight and Obesity Prevention Committee, investigating solutions for childhood obesity. As we combed through a huge stack of studies, the conclusion at the time was that there were no viable solutions.

In 2000, I began working on the frontline of the obesity epidemic at a local community clinic in Huntington Beach, California, and became aware of the day-to-day barriers that my patients were facing. We started by seeing one child at a time, one family at a time, learning about their individual stories and challenges. One family lived in fear in a home where they were told to stay in their rooms and keep quiet. They were not even allowed access to the kitchen. Another lived in a garage with no refrigerator. Others dealt with the stress of sick or disabled family members and were eating nothing but fast food because of time constraints. The concept of developing healthy habits was a dream and an unattainable luxury because these families were in survival mode, just trying to get through the day.

All of these families were tough cases, and all of them required me and my team to piece together what was going on in their homes to determine how best to support them. My compassionate team worked closely with these families, stepping into their shoes and figuring out their barriers and constraints in order to find solutions. For the family living in the garage, we helped find more suitable housing, and my team even found a way to get a refrigerator donated to them.

My team and I have also learned that making subtle changes to the way we approach feeding a child and the psychology with which we approach them about food can make all the difference in the world. For instance, portion control creates more psychological harm than physical good. Maybe a few children will have short-term success with portion control, but the majority will end up with a lifetime of dysfunctional relationships with food—in the same way that intimidation tactics and shaming lead to detrimental results.

I wish I had been Jon Gabriel's doctor when he was young. His story at "fat camp" is a perfect example of a food-restriction philosophy leading to food insecurity, obsession, binging, hoarding, and hiding. His story exemplifies how diets, "diet foods," and other food-related gimmicks don't work. We need to focus on nourishing and supporting our children, not just on calories and diets.

I think of myself as a doctor of community medicine. We are a different breed. We find ways to diagnose illnesses without expensive tests or access to specialists; we consider not just the diagnosis and treatment, but also whether or not the family can execute the plan we create for them. Just because we write a prescription doesn't mean it will get filled—often due to transportation issues or because the family just can't make it to the pharmacy. I remember running into one patient's mom in the hallway at our local hospital. She was crying because she couldn't decide if she should pay to fill her child's asthma medication or pay the electric bill. Another mother's son had horrible diarrhea, and she had to choose whether to use their money for diapers or Pedialyte.

So, how the heck was I going to get these families, who were underinsured, overstressed, and just trying to survive the day-to-day struggles of profound poverty, to change their lifestyles so their children could live healthfully? I wanted these children to have good nutrition, to exercise, excel in school, and grow up to be happy, healthy, successful adults—but their families were scrounging for basic resources like food, shelter, diapers, and clothes.

Early in my career, I had two patients with severe cases of childhood obesity. These two individuals still inspire me to spring out of bed every morning and work with a smile on my face.

I don't remember why Sam came to the clinic initially. I think he had a sore throat. He was twelve years old and weighed 275 pounds. It was quite clear to me that his throat was the least of his problems. In addition to his obvious weight issue, I could also see blackening on the skin of his neck, a sign of insulin resistance called *acanthosis nigricans*, a pre-diabetic condition.

I showed it to his mom. She said, "Oh no, that's from the sun and dirt. He doesn't wash his neck enough." So I said, "Okay, well then let's look under his armpit," because acanthosis nigricans not only shows up as darkening on the neck, but it can also appear in the armpits or in the skin around the waist, just below the navel.

We looked at one of his armpits. Now, armpits are supposed to be as pale as a baby's backside, but Sam's were almost black. And the skin around his waist was the same. These were sure signs of the disease. When I told his mom this, her eyes widened as she explained that his grandpa had diabetes. I now had her full attention.

I ordered some blood tests, but I already knew what the results would be because they were written on his skin. When your sugars are chronically high, over time, they will make the melanocytes, the pigment producing cells in the skin, express themselves and cause skin darkening. Sam was already starting to show signs of type 2 diabetes. Diabetes is a problem with your body that causes blood glucose (sugar) levels to rise higher than normal.

Now, it's one thing to get type 2 diabetes when you're seventy or eighty—by that age you don't really live long enough to suffer the major consequences. But if he kept going in the direction he was headed, Sam would be at risk for all sorts of terrible, and sometimes even life-threatening, complications as an adult, such as kidney failure, amputations, and blindness. Sam needed a new path in life, and he needed it immediately.

It was only then that I discovered there were very few childhood obesity specialists available, particularly for the poor. After calling all my associates, I realized that childhood obesity just wasn't on many people's radar. In fact, when I was at medical school, they only gave us one lecture on obesity, and it was based on one adult patient who weighed 500 pounds. After the lecture, we asked the patient questions, but no one even thought to ask about his childhood or if he had children who might also have weight issues. Obesity was presented specifically as an adult-only problem.

Confronted with Sam and his potentially life-threatening condition, I explained diabetes to him and his mom. I talked to them about heart disease too, and they really listened. And I decided that I was going to have to do whatever I could to help this kid.

"We're going to work together on this, all of us," I said. "Let's see how we can make the food at home healthier, find ways to get Sam to a healthier weight, and get him off this diabetes train." Having no formal training in childhood obesity, I had to wing it, but being at the community clinic, I was used to making things happen without resources. So, not only was I his pediatrician, but I also became his dietician, fitness trainer, and social worker.

One thing I knew from my research and past experience was that the traditional calorie-restriction approach does not work in the long-term. Calorie restriction and deprivation create a feeling of food scarcity for children and causes a mentality of hoarding, hiding, and binging, as evidenced by Jon's fat-camp experience. Children who do this are not rebelling. They become food insecure and react like a prisoner in a concentration camp, wondering if the next meal will come and whether it will be enough. So, rather than following the traditional diet approach, we found ways to offer Sam as many healthy choices as possible and to limit the availability of unhealthy foods.

Sam's mom was great. She got it. After our conversation, it was like a light went on in her head. She realized that diabetes was right around the corner for her son, and she realized the seriousness of the issue and the urgency in dealing with it. They came for multiple visits and follow-ups over the next nine months, and we got the junk food, soda, and other sugary drinks (including 100 percent fruit juice) out of the house—actually saving them money on their grocery bill. She served fruits and vegetables with most meals and snacks. She was motivated. She lost weight, the whole family became healthier, and Sam lost 95 pounds in nine months. Ultimately, Sam did well, and as a reward, I took him to dinner and a hockey game.

Right around this same time, I also met Eddy. He was the first patient I ever had come into the clinic to deal specifically with obesity. Here was a seventeen-year-old kid weighing in at 295 pounds, and like Sam, he was showing extensive signs of acanthosis nigricans, and he had no medical insurance. By working with Eddy in the same way that had I worked with Sam, we managed to turn things around quickly. Eddy lost 100 pounds over a nine-month period.

That's when I knew my calling: treating childhood obesity. The problem was grave, and the number of obese children was increasing. I made a commitment to help prevent obesity through education and guidance, and to stamp out this horrible, misunderstood epidemic, knowing full well that there were no proven methods—particularly diets—available for treating childhood obesity.

I knew that from then on I needed to immerse myself in my patients' plights while I treated them in order to learn as much as I could from them. I also began to document and evaluate my patients through statistics, to prove that our successes weren't anecdotal, but that our work was actually effective.

Our data is comprehensive and sound, and we have been evaluating our programs since 2008. We have statistically significant results so far, but even though the data we have collected over the past five years looks good (amazing, in fact, with 84 percent of our patients improving their body mass index (BMI) percentile in 2012 and 2013), the scientist in me wants to see how all this will pan out over the next fifty years. Will my patients maintain a healthy weight? Will their younger siblings be healthier than they would have been otherwise? How about their children?

As a practicing community pediatrician, I am deep in the trenches of the childhood obesity epidemic. On a regular basis, I see that many of the things we do can't be measured and don't add up into neat statistics. But my amazing team and I have put together some basic premises that seem to be the most effective way to combat this very misunderstood, yet very manageable, disease.

Now, after over a dozen years of experience, I feel like my team and I have come up with a practical formula to help families dealing with childhood obesity. Yet, the scientist in me has to live with the fact that, no, I don't have fifty years of data. But then again, neither does the rest of the scientific community, and it feels like a sin to wait to get the message out. I am already teaching other medical providers who are begging for direction, and I feel like I need to get the word out to everyone struggling with this epidemic, including you.

I don't want the overweight children of today, and you, the parents and caregivers of these children, to wait fifty years to confirm the effectiveness of what we are doing now. We're in too much of a crisis to wait another second. And to be honest, the tactics we use are not strong medications, fancy procedures, or aggressive treatments. The tactics we use are family based; they bring families closer together and dispel myths about what foods are considered healthy. For more than twelve years, I've dedicated my career to treating childhood obesity, and now I am here to help you and your child on your road to a healthy, happy life.

Introduction:
When We See Kids Today

As parents, we try to understand what's happening in our children's worlds. We try to understand their thoughts, feelings, activities, foods, and stresses, their responses to life and the decisions they make—we especially try to understand how they feel about themselves and what they feel they can achieve.

Children are subjected to enormous stresses and pressures at school from both adults and from each other, as well as powerfully induced false beliefs about their bodies from social marketing and the media.

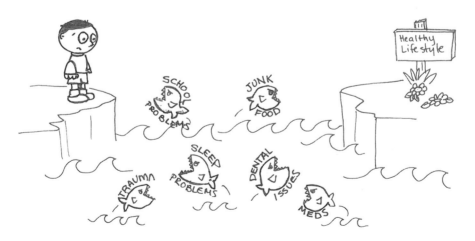

These stresses and pressures, these messages and beliefs, all contribute to weight gain in children. The usual methods of blaming, shaming, and punishment only add to these negative forces and make things even worse. Unfortunately, we're applying a broken paradigm of behavior modification and calorie control to kids. It didn't work in the fat camp days, and it won't work today, tomorrow, or ever.

There's underlying shaming going on. Overtly, peers and professionals use emotional bullying and bad-mouthing. Covertly, there's an understanding that children, and their parents, are not doing their part in controlling their weight. This false belief, that it's either the parent's or the child's fault, is pervasive and unquestioned.

Jon knows one woman who won't carry a picture of her granddaughter in her wallet because the little girl is overweight. She carries a picture of the child from four years ago before she gained the weight. What this lady doesn't get is that her granddaughter has no control over a body that wants to gain weight. Would she carry a picture of her grandchild if she had asthma or if she was in a wheelchair? Of course she would. What's the difference between having asthma and having obesity? We manage the asthma because we recognize that there are forces that trigger an asthmatic response, and we know that it's not the child's fault.

Sadly, we're *ashamed* of the kid who is overweight because we fail to recognize that there are forces that trigger an obesity response, and we're under the false impression that overweight kids can do something about their obesity, but they don't because of their own laziness, willfulness, rebellion, sheer stubbornness, or any other number of "character flaws." The whole situation gets even worse when we blame ourselves for their "failings"—believing their "lack of discipline" or "self-control" is our fault because we are bad parents. But how on earth can we reasonably expect a child to do something, how can we expect ourselves to do something, about a situation like weight gain that society as a whole is clueless about?

Even more disturbing is that the bullying is much worse within peer groups. Back in 2002, when Jon was at his heaviest, he was in an office waiting room, sitting across from a slender ten-year-old boy, whose father was nearby talking to the receptionist. At first, Jon felt bad for the kid, thinking he maybe had some rare form of Tourette's syndrome because he had a kind of convulsive jerking twitch. He would jerk his head while making snorting noises.

As he and his father were leaving, he looked Jon in the eye and made the same snorting noise. That's when it became clear that there was nothing wrong with this kid; he was just making pig noises. He felt the need to acknowledge Jon's weight by snorting like a pig in front of his father and a room full of professionals. His father didn't seem to mind at all.

One can't help but wonder: if this kid felt the need to make fun of a man twice his height and five times his weight, what on earth was he saying to his overweight peers at the park? If it was okay for him to abuse fat adults, what was he doing to fat kids, and maybe still doing to others today? He and others who make fun of overweight people are setting up their peers to think that they're losers at everything—traumatizing them for life.

This is what it's like to suffer the cruel and constant indignity of being an overweight child. If the child in Jon's story was indeed treating his peers like he treated Jon, he was destroying lives on a daily basis. But was it really the kid's fault? His father seemed to have learned, seemingly like everyone else, that people are fat because they're weak and lazy and just eat too much. So the kid, in turn, had learned that fat people are fair game. He'd learned that attitude from his father, and why should his father think anything different, when doctors, medical schools, and policy makers are still telling us that obesity is caused by eating too much and the solution is to just "eat less"—calories in and calories out, nothing more? If all this blaming, shaming, and abuse is going to stop, we need to look at the facts, even though they haven't made it into mainstream wisdom yet. We need to be a different type of parent, the type who knows and understands both intuitively and intellectually that there's more going on than simply calories in and calories out, that our children are not weak or lazy or overindulgent. There are other factors at play, and we need to look at those factors. We need to see how flawed and broken the current dieting paradigm is and fix it ourselves.

We figure that you're already a different sort of parent.

That is why you're reading this book in the first place.

It's no fun being an overweight kid, especially in a world where people want to humiliate you all the time, as if somehow you can be humiliated into thinness.

In this book, we want to help you take your child from a place of frustration, failure, and hopeless despair to a place of confidence, success, and renewed passion. By reducing stress in your children's social and physical surroundings, by nourishing their bodies and spirits, and by providing an environment that is safe, loving, and supportive, removing all the forces that are making and keeping our kids fat, we can make a world of difference to them. The result will be healthier, happier, and more successful children who grow up to be healthier, happier, and more successful adults.

We want to create a clear path for you and your family as you learn to understand and implement the proper psychology of feeding children. We want to educate you on nutrition (without gimmicks). We want to help you deepen your bonds with your children and find strategies for dealing with the inevitable stresses that all families experience (not just those living in poverty), and as a result, help your child regain a natural, normal velocity of growth and eventually a healthy weight, while also gaining energy, improving concentration and focus, and increasing confidence, security, and happiness.

That's our commitment to you.

Currently, childhood obesity affects one in three American kids and teens.[1] Childhood obesity is now the number one health concern among parents in the United States, topping drug abuse and smoking.[2]

The epidemic of childhood obesity is a symptom of a changed world: greater technology, more processed food sources, sedentary behaviors, marketing ploys, sleep deprivation, stress, troubled finances, and the de-emphasis of the family unit—we are all just a little caught up in it.

There is a reason that obesity is the number one health concern for parents. Obesity in youth is associated with a host of immediate and long-term medical problems, including heart disease, type 2 diabetes, liver failure, stroke, asthma, and cancer.[3,4] Just as concerning are the psychological complications that overweight youth face. Obese children are four times more likely to have impaired ability to learn and are much more likely to be depressed or anxious, and are more likely to have the quality of life comparable to children in chemotherapy or who have been diagnosed with cancer.[5]

In addition to the immediate health risks, obese children are more likely to become obese adults. The severity of this issue is best described by former Surgeon General Richard Carmona, who explained, "Because of the increasing rates of obesity, unhealthy eating habits and physical inactivity, we may see the first generation that will be less healthy and have a shorter life expectancy than their parents."[6]

No one wants to be unhealthy, and even more so, they don't want their children to be unhealthy. In fact, deep down, we desire good health for ourselves but especially for our children. Yet, it is amazing how many put little or no thought into achieving health for themselves or for their children. Meanwhile, many others are preoccupied with it, to the point of being obsessed. Those at either extreme are not necessarily at fault. We know that most parents fall somewhere in between. But what is more appalling is the amount of confusion and misinformation about how to optimize our health, particularly when it comes to weight loss for kids. This predicament of how to help our kids maintain a healthy weight and balanced life is a challenge not only for parents, but for healthcare professionals as well.

Perhaps you, like many parents out there, have already been trying to help your child lose weight, but it hasn't been working, and instead, it's adding more stress to your lives—and your relationship with your child is suffering as a result.

The goal of this book is to give you practical, rewarding, doable guidance that will help your child and make your whole family healthier in the process. Very simple changes can have a dramatic impact on your child's health, and tough challenges can be overcome, as well, by using the principles that we lay out in this book.

In the following chapters, we will show you how to achieve what you likely want most: for your children to be healthy. We will show you how to achieve this by helping you succeed in areas that are likely at the very heart of your purpose in life: to be closer to your child, enjoy meals together, be healthier yourself, and build a strong foundation for your child's life, their children's lives, and so on.

The beauty of our philosophy is that it promotes stronger relationships, playtime, and natural foods—essentially reverting back to basic concepts we have all gotten away from in this modern world. We are excited to help you learn to enjoy family meals and for your whole family to become healthier.

We are both deeply committed to helping solve this very tragic, yet preventable, epidemic. We need to get the word out to change the world's inaccurate, detrimental view toward obesity, diets, and the psychology of feeding children.

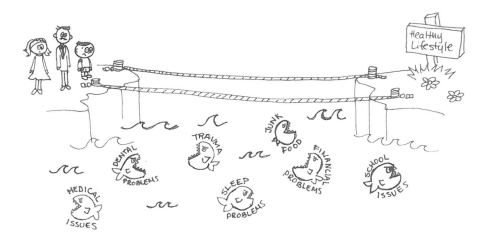

1

The Flawed Diet Approach

"You want to lose weight? Just eat less."

We're sure you've heard comments like these all your life, spoken in a well-intentioned manner. This is the conventional wisdom that we've all grown up with and that many physicians use to treat childhood obesity today. But these days this conventional wisdom is being very heavily scrutinized. Why? Simply put, it doesn't work. Let's face it, if diets worked, there'd be one popular diet, maybe two. Everyone would go on them. Everyone would lose weight, and that would be the end of it. There wouldn't be hundreds of diets all operating on the premise that you can somehow force yourself to lose weight and keep it off. The problem is that the very premise on which all of these calorie-restrictive diets are based is flawed.

A great many healthcare providers still subscribe to the old idea that obesity is simply the result of too many calories in and not enough calories out. If you subscribe to this faulty logic, then it's only natural to advise people to just eat less and restrict their calories. This is what dieting is: the expectation that fewer calories in will automatically make your body use the calories stored in your fat cells, and then as those calories get used, all that extra fat will disappear, revealing the slimmer, trimmer you underneath.

The other expectation is that once your body has lost all this excess fat, it will automatically want to stay that way forever and your hunger levels will adjust to help you maintain a new, slimmer, trimmer you for the rest of your life. Unfortunately, our bodies just aren't designed like that. The reality is that restrictive dieting doesn't work to create sustainable, permanent weight loss. Our bodies' intricately designed survival mechanisms work in exactly the opposite way than they're "supposed to" according to popular diet theory. There's now plenty of evidence to demonstrate that diets are based on this flawed premise.

In April 2007, *American Psychologist*, the journal of the American Psychological Association, reported findings from a study conducted by the University of California, Los Angeles.[1] The UCLA team analyzed thirty-one long-term studies on the relationship between dieting and weight loss. The fundamental question they sought to answer: will you lose weight and keep it off if you diet?

The answer: probably not.

"You can initially lose 5 to 10 percent of your weight on any number of diets, but then the weight comes back," said Traci Mann, UCLA associate professor of psychology and lead author of the study. "We found that the majority of people regained all the weight, plus more. Sustained weight loss was found only in a small minority of participants, while complete weight regain was found in the majority. *Diets do not lead to sustained weight loss or health benefits for the majority of people* [our italics]."[2] Remember that the UCLA study was the result of examining thirty-one other studies, and the overwhelming conclusion was, and still is, that diets don't work.

Many people know this from their own experience. And yet, there's still a huge dieting industry and large numbers of healthcare professionals who believe that diets are the answer. Before you can really deal with the weight issue in anyone, including your children, you need a new way of looking at the world. You need a new paradigm.

- **Paradigm Shift No. 1:** Not only do diets not work, but dieting makes your body *want* to gain weight.

We've been hard-pressed to find studies that look into the long-term effects of dieting on children, but if diets don't work long-term for adults, why would they work for kids? Remember that our bodies, and our children's bodies, are not independent of our brains. Dieting creates hormonal changes that affect every part of our bodies, including our brains.

There is now an increasing body of scientific evidence showing how these hormonal changes conspire against you. An April 2012 article in the UK newspaper *The Daily Mail* reported:

For the 25 per cent of Britons trying to lose weight at any one time: our basic human biology is the greatest enemy of committed slimmers.

Researchers, including Joseph Proietto, a professor of medicine at the University of Melbourne, have uncovered one of the main possible reasons. Two years ago, his team recruited fifty obese men and women, and coached them through eight weeks of an extreme 500-to-550-calories-a-day diet (a quarter of the normal intake for women).

At the end, the dieters lost an average of 30 pounds. Proietto's team then spent a year giving them counseling support to stick to healthy eating habits. But during this time, the dieters regained an average of 11 pounds. *They also reported feeling far hungrier and more preoccupied with food than before losing weight* [our italics].

As the researchers reported in *The New England Journal of Medicine*, the volunteers' hormones were working overtime, making them react as though they were starving and in need of weight gain. Their levels of an appetite-stimulating hormone, ghrelin, were about 20 per cent higher than at the start of the study. Meanwhile, their levels of an appetite-suppressing hormone, peptide YY, were unusually low.

Furthermore, levels of leptin, a hormone that suppresses hunger and raises the metabolic rate, also remained lower than expected. Proietto describes this effect as:

"'a coordinated defense mechanism with multiple components all directed toward making us put on weight.' In other words, *the body had launched a backlash against dieting* [our italics]."

Research has revealed that about eight weeks into the dieting process an effect kicks in, resetting your metabolism to function on fewer calories, storing extra calories as fat and that this effect can last for years.[3]

The tragedy is that dieters blame their failures on themselves, pointing the finger at their own imagined inadequacy, or failing that, they blame their genes. More relevant to our subject is that children who have been put on diets have the real potential to grow up with guilt and, even worse, a dysfunctional relationship with food that may last for the rest of their lives. And yes, genetics does play some role, but we can't blame *only* our genes anymore either. The *Tampa Bay Times* cites a Finnish study that investigated dieting in genetically identical twins. What makes us fat? Is it our genes or the dieting? According to Dr. Kirsi Pietilainen, lead author of the study, it's the dieting: "They found that identical twins who attempt to lose weight tend to end up heavier than their non-dieting siblings."[4]

We live in a world where so much of our social life and social identity revolves around food. In the *Tampa Bay Times* article, actor Jonah Hill describes his struggle with his weight. Hill has appeared in several major motion pictures, such as *Superbad* and *The Wolf of Wall Street*, and he says he's had his own struggle with yo-yo dieting. "Gaining fifty pounds would probably be more fun than losing fifty pounds for a part."[5]

Many people would agree, so denying ourselves or our children the pleasure of food becomes an exercise in discipline and denial, and our inability to succeed becomes evidence of our lack, or our children's lack, of moral fiber. We end up attributing our weight-loss failures to flaws in our personality, and we end up with a world full of committed dieters who fail and who don't realize that the real problem is not them but the diet process, what we call the Flawed Diet Approach.

But blaming the victims of the Flawed Diet Approach continues, and if adults blame themselves, how much worse is it for kids? We need a paradigm shift.

It's the approach that's at fault, not the person.

From a purely attitudinal point of view, diets create a food-scarcity and a hoarding mentality in children, and they start to fight us, even as we're trying to help them. When this happens, we tend to label them as "rebellious" or "difficult," but in truth they're not rebelling. They're simply responding to insecurities they've formed around food. They're asking themselves, *Will I get enough food?*—because the dieting process itself alters their brain chemistry, making them want to eat more. Thus, their brain chemistry conspires with their natural desire to survive. This creates a vicious cycle—biochemistry reinforcing behavior—and your child's body and brain fight at a chemical level. The result:

Dieting creates an unhealthy relationship between food, self-image, and self-esteem that can become lifelong and ultimately life-threatening.

Childhood dieting often sets the stage for a lifetime of problems. An ever-increasing number of professionals have learned through their own journeys that diets don't work. In his blog for *The Huffington Post*, psychotherapist William Anderson even went so far as to say that he "didn't have a weight problem until after the first diet."[6] At the age of seven, he was put on calorie restriction because he was a "bit husky," and that's when all the problems started:

Having the freedom to eat whatever I wanted was not an important issue before the diet, but it sure was after. It's the same with treats. *Cookies, cakes and candies became highly valued needs, much more important to me than they were before the diet* [our italics]. Eating freely became the most important thing in my day, something that I soon did at every opportunity. I became an overeater, worsening with each diet. I became the "fat kid," the heaviest kid at the weigh-ins at school, 225 pounds at 5 feet 6 inches in junior high, and over 300 as an adult, until my early thirties.[7]

We can't overemphasize how important the issue of mindset is to the success or failure of weight loss. Even the *perception* of being fat is important. An August 2012 article in *US News & World Report*, titled "The Diet Mentality Paradox: Why Dieting Can Make You Fat," cites a study published in the *Journal of Obesity* that reported:

Normal-weight teenagers were more likely to be overweight ten years later if they thought of themselves as overweight to begin with. This is not a new observation. Earlier studies, such as one published in the *Journal of the American Dietetic Association*, identified the same problem: kids who feel fat are more likely to be fat years later.[8]

Consider the implications of this. Even if kids who have normal weight think that they're obese, they'll become obese. Even beyond the hormones and the chemistry, the Flawed Diet Approach encourages the creation of the *diet mentality*. As the article maintains, "The diet mentality is created by the act of dieting itself, and is basically a self-destructive pattern of thinking and behaving."[9]

Have you ever gone to dinner with a friend who ordered French fries, wings, beer-battered rings, and pie a la mode because tomorrow was the start of her diet? Or have you ever heard someone say they were going for ice cream because they "earned" it by going to the gym that day? Maybe you've been on a diet and found yourself dreaming about foods that were now restricted, when you never even gave them a second thought in the past. This is the diet mentality at work. Dieting, as the *US News & World Report* article also reports, creates a perfect storm of restrictive eating patterns that cannot be maintained, along with feelings of shame and guilt. Eventually, most dieters fall off the wagon, which leads to weight gain.[10]

If this is the case for adults, how much more common will it be with children, who often don't have the same mental, emotional, and physical resources to cope with the effects of a diet? Dr. Patricia had an 80-pound, three-year-old boy, Brady (whose weight should have been around 33 pounds at that age), come to see her, and he was carrying around a measuring cup. She thought it was so cute, that maybe he wanted to be a chef when he grew up. But she came to discover that Brady had previously seen a registered dietitian, who said he could only eat carbs in a quantity that would fit into the cup, so he was carrying it with him everywhere he went in anticipation of his next portion—or should we say *ration*—of food. Not only did this restrictive way of portion control make him become completely insecure about food, but he also proceeded to escalate from overweight to obese.

He was finally referred to Dr. Patricia's program, where they were able to undo the damage. The parents were grateful and relieved when Dr. Patricia explained what was going on with their child. At some level, they knew they had been going in the wrong direction.

Consider for a moment what children in this position must be feeling. What are they thinking about? How often are they wondering when they can get their ice cream, cookies, or candy? How often are they thinking about how they can get the food that they want, the food that their bodies' hormones are telling them they want, despite what the grown-ups are saying? And how many hours are their developing minds fixated on what they are going to eat? How much of this fixation are they going to take with them into adulthood, where it will lead to an ongoing dysfunctional relationship with food?

The conspiracy between biology and psychology, the feelings of disempowerment, and the subsequent dysfunctional relationship with food that dieting creates, especially in an overweight child, are the main reasons we need a weight-loss approach for our children that addresses both the body and the mind.

We need to find ways to get our kids' bodies to switch back to a healthier metabolism for optimal growth, strategies for nourishing them both physically and emotionally, and techniques to make them feel more empowered and self-reliant, so that they won't be fighting *you*, because they won't be fighting *themselves*. You, your child, and your child's biology need to be on the same team, with the same goals and the same level of enthusiasm. We can accomplish this far more easily if we first make the paradigm shift away from forced restriction and focus more on addressing the real issues. Dieting will not lead to long-term, sustainable weight loss. It just doesn't work that way.

The principles outlined in this book are not a diet. They involve appropriate nutrition and psychology that will benefit everyone, of every size, in your family. Our intention is to give you tools to overcome the barriers to good health that are in your home, so that you can create a healthy environment, make mealtimes more enjoyable, and address any problems concerning stress, poor nutrition, or unhealthy growth—for everyone.

Overcoming barriers with these principles will help normalize your child's growth. This does not always mean that they will lose weight, since children are growing. In fact, if they stop or slow down weight gain while continuing to grow, they will get leaner. But, please refrain from getting the child on a scale to monitor success because we don't want them to become anxious or obsessed about their weight, feel like they're on a diet, or feel pressured one way or another. We want kids to be kids, and if they are served a variety of healthy foods in a psychologically sound way and in a safe environment, they will get healthier and more fit in a natural and sustainable way.

If dieting isn't the cure for obesity, what is? Before we answer that question, we have to understand the real reasons your child, or anyone else for that matter, gains excessive weight, because if we don't understand the real causes, we can't come up with the real answers.

Calories are only one of many factors contributing to weight gain.

2

The Real Reasons Our Kids Are Overweight

The biggest problem with the old calories in and calories out diet paradigm is that we never end up asking the real questions about why a child is overweight in the first place. If weight gain is just a question of eating too much, then obviously the solution is simply to eat less. But if, as we have seen, eating too much, craving the wrong foods, or being overly sedentary are just the symptoms of a real, fundamental, underlying cause, then it begs the question:

What is the *real* cause of weight gain?

This leads us to our second major paradigm shift.

- **Paradigm Shift No. 2:** Children don't gain weight just because they eat too much. In fact, our bodies have a survival mechanism that causes us to gain weight. We call it a Famine And Temperature (FAT) Switch or FAT Program, and when this switch is activated, our bodies literally transform themselves into fat storage machines. The way to solve your child's weight problem is to find out what's activating the FAT switch and then to turn it off.

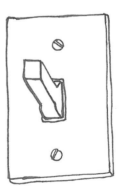

We realize this paradigm shift runs counter to a lot of what people tell you about obesity, and it even runs counter to "common sense," but people don't become overweight just because they eat too much.

If your FAT switch is on, you will gain weight even if you eat less than people of normal weight do.

Fat, like everything else, isn't all bad. Fat is essential to life. The first thing that we need to understand is that our bodies have one primary, overriding goal, and that is *to survive*. Our bodies will do whatever it takes to keep us safe and alive.

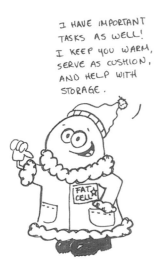

I HAVE IMPORTANT TASKS AS WELL! I KEEP YOU WARM, SERVE AS CUSHION, AND HELP WITH STORAGE.

Fat is essential, just like oxygen, water, and sleep, but just like you must have the right amount of oxygen, water, and sleep, you also must have the right amount of fat. For example, our bodies always make sure we get enough oxygen—the key word here being *enough*.

If we breathe too fast for too long, we hyperventilate and pass out (and subsequently restore a normal breathing pattern). And then there is the problem of not getting enough air. If we start to asphyxiate because we're choking or drowning, our brains and bodies immediately go into survival mode and turn on a kind of "oxygen switch," and we experience an overwhelming urge to breathe.

This switch is so powerful it overrides everything, even conscious thought.

If you've ever seen anyone choking and witnessed that person thrashing around as they try to get air, you'll know what we mean. When the air finally comes, they experience uncontrollable gasping, until their cells get enough oxygen. When a survival switch is on, it doesn't just flood our awareness with a compulsion to act, it literally takes over, and our behavior changes to get us out of the crisis. This switch is so powerful it even operates in our sleep. If we have interrupted oxygen during sleep, we actually wake up temporarily—this is part of a condition called *sleep apnea*, which has its own connection to obesity. We'll explore that more in chapter 6.

Speaking of sleep, a similar thing happens when we're sleep deprived. As everybody knows, if you've gone a night without sleeping, you will be tired all the time and fighting the urge to sleep nonstop. If you go two nights without sleep, it becomes almost impossible to avoid nodding off, because getting enough sleep is also vital to our survival. There's a great scene in the 1950s classic science-fiction movie *Invasion of the Body Snatchers* that illustrates this point beautifully.

A couple of twentysomethings have figured out that, while they sleep, the people in their town are being replaced by aliens that grow in pods, and the aliens are trying to take over Earth. Our heroes struggle and struggle not to fall asleep, because they know if they do, they're going to be totally doomed. But try as they might, after days of staying awake, they finally succumb and . . . zzzz.

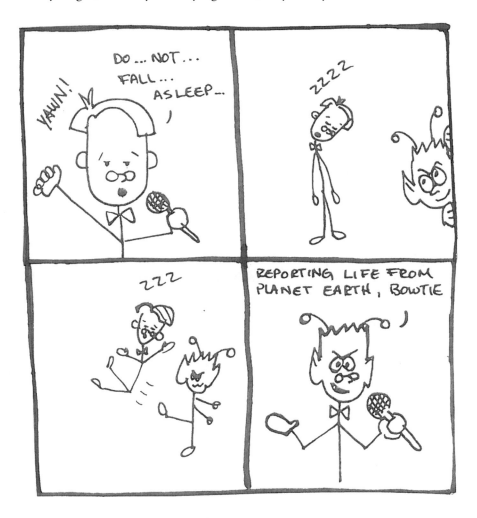

In the next scene, we see our brave, young twentysomethings staring glassy-eyed and doing a zombie walk, along with a whole bunch of other glassy-eyed, staring zombies, and we know what's happened. So why did these characters in *Invasion of the Body Snatchers* fall asleep, even though in doing so they were going to be murdered and then replaced by homicidal aliens?

They fell asleep because no amount of willpower can stop you from falling asleep when your body forces you to. Our bodies' survival switches are too powerful, too compelling to be overridden by something as feeble as this mythical "willpower" that we're all supposed to have. This "failure of willpower" doesn't make us weak; it simply means that when our survival is at stake, our bodies are completely in charge, and any and all illusions that we are in control fly out the window. You can't override a survival switch through "willpower," and your child can't either.

What's true of the need for oxygen and sleep is also true for fat. Just like you, your child's body has an optimum set point for what it thinks is a healthy level of fat for its age and environment. A little bit of fat is healthy. A lot is not. There's a healthy range for all of us, and our body will always try to maintain that healthy weight.

So what happens in the overweight body? Why do people get fat even when they're "on a diet" and eating less than normal?

Imagine for a second that your brain thought that you had zero fat on your body. Regardless of the real situation, if your brain *thought* that it had zero body fat, what do you think it would do?

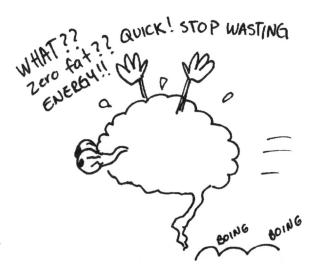

Your body would immediately go into crisis mode.[1] It would turn on a FAT switch, compelling you to put on as much fat as you could, as quickly as you possibly could. The same survival mechanisms that force you to breathe and force you to sleep would also force you to eat. You'd become insatiably hungry, you'd crave the most fattening foods possible, and you might even become tired and lethargic in order to conserve energy. Your entire outlook would tend to become focused on food, and your body would compellingly, overwhelmingly want to get fatter.

Like every other survival crisis situation, the switch would be on, and you would have no more power to override it than you would have to overcome the urge to breathe if you held your breath for too long, or the urge to sleep if you stayed awake for too long.

You would be powerless, *willpower-less*, in the face of your body's need to become fatter.

Now imagine that you were carrying 50 or 100 or even 200 extra pounds of fat, and your brain *still* thought that there was no fat on your body. Regardless of the reality, if for whatever reason, your brain thought that you had no fat on your body, the result would still be the same. You'd be insatiably hungry, and you'd be craving the sweetest and most fattening foods possible. This scenario is real. This misreading of the body's true amount of fat is caused by something called *leptin resistance* and is part of a series of hormonal changes that can take place when your children's bodies accidently turn on their FAT switch. It is almost always the case that our bodies mistakenly activate this FAT switch *not* because of famine-induced starvation, but rather, because of some kind of mental, physical, or emotional stress.

One of the side effects of leptin resistance is that our taste buds change and become less sensitive to sweet food, so it takes sweeter foods to satisfy us. A September 2012 article in *Time*, states:

> German researchers report that obese kids have less sensitive taste buds than their normal weight peers, and may therefore eat more food to get the same flavor sensation.
>
> The researchers looked at 193 healthy children aged 6 to 18. Roughly half the kids were normal weight and half were obese. For the study, researchers placed 22 taste strips on the children's tongues, representing each of the five types of taste—sweet, sour, salty, umami (savory) and bitter—at four levels of intensity, as well as two blank strips. The participants were asked to identify each of the tastes, and also rank each taste strip's level of intensity.
>
> Each taste was assigned a score, with the maximum score for identifying all five types of taste at the four different intensity levels adding up to 20. Obese kids had a significantly more difficult time

distinguishing between tastes, resulting in an average score of 12.6, compared with an average of just over 14 for the normal weight kids [that's a 10 percent difference we note]. As most kids got older, their ability to differentiate between taste sensations improved, *but not among obese children* [our italics]. And although all the kids correctly identified the different sweetness intensity levels, *obese kids rated most of the higher-intensity taste strips as weaker than did the normal weight kids* [our italics].[2]

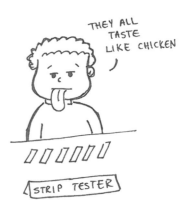

Some other symptoms of leptin and insulin resistance are:

• Insatiable hunger
• Incessant craving of sweet or calorie-dense foods
• Chronic fatigue or lethargy

Just as telling someone who hasn't slept in two days to stay awake won't work, no matter how much you scream at them, telling a leptin-resistant child to eat less is cruel and futile and promotes a dysfunctional relationship with food. In fact, telling anyone to eat less may trigger food insecurity, hoarding, and hiding.

Dr. Jeffrey Friedman discovered the leptin hormone in the early nineties, and he understood the mechanisms that conspire to force you to gain weight when you're leptin resistant. Dr. Friedman says, "obesity cannot be ascribed simply to a breakdown in willpower," and we have got to "resist the impulse to assign blame."[3] If, for whatever reason, this FAT switch is on, even though there's no threat of starvation and fat levels are normal or above normal, your child's brain is getting an inaccurate assessment of how much fat is on his body, and in some cases, his brain may think that he's carrying zero fat, when in fact he may be morbidly obese.

Remember this really important point. What do all the survival switches have in common? They are all responses to stresses: the stress of not having enough oxygen, sleep, or body fat. There are other survival switches too, which are just as involuntary and compelling, like the switch that forces you to shiver when you get too cold or the uncontrollable thirst caused by dehydration—but you get the picture.

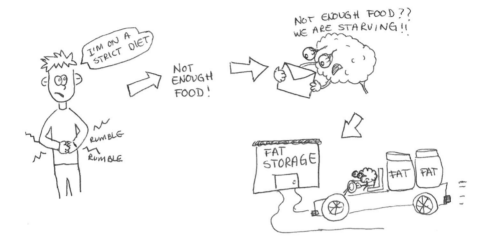

If we look at obesity as a survival switch issue, then certain confusing things suddenly become clear. Obviously, dieting can turn *on* the FAT switch, although it's only really obvious once you make the paradigm shift. Why does dieting turn on the FAT switch? Because dieting sends a message to the body that there isn't enough food available.

Our bodies are built to respond to starvation, or the threat of starvation, by activating this FAT switch. That's the very reason we have a FAT switch in the first place, to protect us from famine. And dieting is an artificial famine. If the FAT switch is already on because some malfunction in the body has confused it, this means that our bodies are already acting under the mistaken notion that we are in a famine, that there's not enough to eat, and that we're starving. It doesn't matter that we live a world full of all-you-can-eat, cheaply available, empty calories. And it also doesn't matter that you or your child might have tremendous excess reserves of fat already. If the body is tricked into activating this FAT switch, it's operating under the false impression that it's starving.

As previously mentioned, FAT stands for Famine And Temperature. In the world that our ancestors lived in for thousands of years, the most appropriate response to famine or low temperatures was for our brains and bodies to turn on the FAT switch and to make us gain weight. Faced with the threat of starving or freezing, our entire way of perceiving the world would change, turning us into fat storage machines in order to ensure our survival. In the natural course of events, as soon as the weather warmed up and there was plenty of food around, our brains would turn off the FAT switch and our bodies would *want* to get thin again.

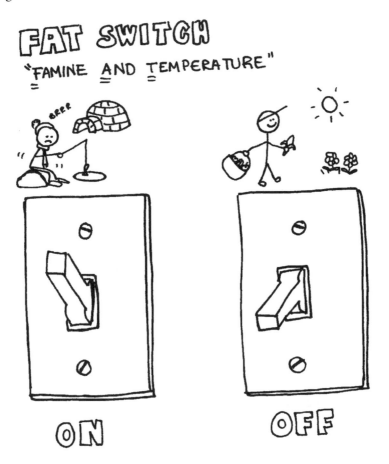

Our bodies would suddenly want to slim down, because as great as fat is for getting us through a famine or a cold winter, it's not such a great idea to keep too much fat on when we don't need it. The FAT switch should turn on naturally and appropriately as a response to stress when there's not enough food to eat or when the weather is too cold, and then turn off again when things get better.

But in today's world, there are many other stressors that can trick your children's bodies—or your own body—into turning on the FAT switch.

The FAT switch creates a different chemical environment in the body. The obese body is a very different body than the normal body, not just because it's obese. It became *chemically different* in order to become obese.

Experientially you'll see that when the FAT switch is on, everything changes—impulses, attitudes, and behaviors—all in the service of turning you or your child's body into a fat storage machine.

When you make the paradigm shift, you realize that people don't become obese because they sit around eating all day or because they're "lazy" and "self-indulgent." They gain weight because their bodies have responded to a particular type of stress, their FAT switch is now on, and their bodies now want to be obese.

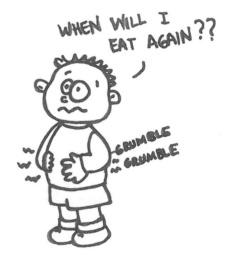

This switch makes them inactive in order to conserve energy so that more energy is available to be turned into fat. This switch also makes them crave food in order to provide more calories that can be turned into fat.

Overeating and inactivity can then be seen as the symptoms, not the cause of weight gain. When the fat switch is on in your child's body, the entire chemical, hormonal, and even neurological environment changes to make the body fat. Even if you're not eating much at all, being forced to eat less reinforces your body's mistaken notion that you're in a famine, and that makes the FAT switch even more active.

Sustainable weight loss is only possible when you address the stresses that turn the switch on in the first place, because you can't fight the FAT switch. The switch is on because, in response to stress, your body, however mistaken it might be, is trying to keep you alive.

When you remove the stresses, you remove the reason the FAT switch is on in the first place. Without the reason for the switch to be on, the brain says, "Great! Crisis over. Sigh of relief. Time to get lean again," and it will turn the switch off, initiating a domino effect of changes that will make your child's body want to get thin again, as quickly and as naturally as possible. When the chemical conditions that caused the survival mechanism finally change, it's almost like the brain says, "Where did all this fat come from?" and in an instant, the brain makes chemical changes throughout the body that cause your child to become less hungry, crave fewer fattening foods, and for their body to speed up its metabolism. The body also becomes very efficient at burning fat. In essence, the whole fat storage mechanism gets reversed. This is the way to lose fat safely and sustainably: by creating a chemical condition in the body that's conducive to effortless weight loss. By removing or modifying the stresses that caused the switch to be on in the first place, weight begins to fall off.

Once the FAT switch is turned off, you will have a different chemistry—a chemistry that wants you to be thin from the inside out and a body that will suddenly become more active; wants to eat less; and actually craves fruit, vegetables, and salads, instead of junk food. So, what modern-world stresses trigger the FAT switch? The short answer is: anything that causes a chemical condition in the body, similar to chronic starvation or cold, is going to turn on the switch.

Common Stresses that Make Our Bodies Hold on to Weight

- Restrictive dieting, because it mimics starvation (portion control in any form or deliberately skipping meals and snacks).
- Nutritional famine, when we're not getting essential elements in our food.
- Processed foods, a variation on the theme of nutritional famine because of the inevitable depletion of nutrients in processing. Processed foods also cause hormonal fluctuations in our bodies that can lead to leptin and insulin resistance.
- Digestion problems, when we're not absorbing essential elements, even if they are in our food.
- Anything that causes chronic, low-grade inflammation, because this causes hormonal changes that can turn on the FAT switch.
- Certain medications, because they alter the body's chemistry.
- Mental or chronic stress, because it can cause chemical changes in our bodies that are similar to the stress of a famine or cold weather.
- Emotional trauma and abuse, as sometimes the body uses weight as a form of protection against emotional trauma and physical and mental abuse.
- Excessive toxins, which can cause chemical and hormonal changes in our body that can activate the FAT switch. This affects the genes and may alter metabolic rates, meaning our bodies hoard calories rather than burn them.[4]

- Sleep apnea and sleep problems, because they elevate cortisol levels, which causes leptin and insulin resistance.
- Chronic dehydration, also a chronic stress that can activate the FAT switch.

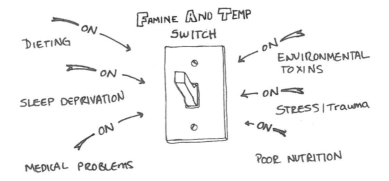

It stands to reason that since you and your child have similar genetics, reside under the same roof, and live in similar physical and economic environments, it's likely that you are experiencing the same stresses, and your bodies are responding to those stresses in similar ways. By now, it should come as no surprise to you that addressing these stressors means not only dealing with an overweight child's body, but it also means dealing with the child's heart and mind too—*the whole child*—and almost inevitably, *the whole family*.

We're going to be giving you lots of information in the coming chapters, along with lots of very practical suggestion and solutions. You'll start to see some common themes in the suggestions we offer you, which will help you make sense of it all. The advice we offer nearly always centers around some form of nourishment—nourishment for your child, nourishment for you, nourishment for you family, and nourishment at every level: physically, mentally, emotionally, and spiritually.

If you have any questions along the way, please contact us at TheGabriel Method.com/FitKids and DrRibasHealthClub.org/FitKids. There, you'll also find lots of yummy recipes and simple practical advice for helping you and your family live fit, healthy, happy lives.

3

Nourish Your Child's Body

Just because you can put something in your mouth and swallow it, that doesn't mean that it's food. Food, real food, is about nutrition—nourishing your child's body with the essential elements that it needs not only to survive, but also to grow and thrive. It follows then that nutritionally poor food doesn't have what it takes to keep a body healthy. The inevitable result of poor nutrition is malnourishment, which can lead to becoming underweight, nutritionally deficient, having Failure to Thrive (FTT) and, ironically, becoming obese.

Here's a question Dr. Patricia always asks the kids she works with: if someone gave you a brand-new Maserati, what would you put in the gas tank?

It is not likely you will get another free car, so you better put the right stuff in it and on it, like good gas in the tank, air in the tires, and a nice outer coat of wax so that it will last for a long time.

Would you ever consider putting soap in your gas tank? A can of soda where your oil would go? Tar on your paint? No, right? Because that would ruin your fabulous new car.

The concept of caring for a car can be transferred into caring for one's body, which helps children quickly understand the importance of nourishing their bodies properly.

The reason we eat is to ingest and assimilate nutrients. Why are we feeding our children foods devoid of these nutrients?

The question is how do you get into the habit of feeding your family healthy foods? Start with these three basic rules:

1. Add fresh fruit or vegetables to all meals and snacks.
2. Serve water to drink instead of juice or other sweetened beverages.
3. Choose the most natural foods for your family to eat (including unprocessed meats and grains).

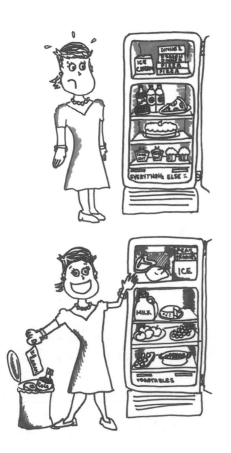

So, the first step to feeding your family healthy foods is emptying your pantry and fridge of nutritionally poor foods. The only way to fill the house with nutritionally dense, healthy foods is to first do some spring-cleaning.

Go and carefully read the food labels in your home right now. It may sound like an arduous task, but keep in mind that if these foods are in your home, they will end up in your children's bodies. You can do a slow approach and choose to stop buying these foods, and eventually they will run out. If that is all you think you can handle, let's start there. But if you can do some purging, that will be the quickest way to meet your family's nutritional needs.

Some foods, like ice cream and cake, seem more obviously bad to many people because of their high sugar content, artificial colors, and other issues, while other foods, like cereal and flavored yogurt, seem healthier than they are due to clever marketing. Also, do not be fooled by natural, healthy foods that sometimes have unnecessary added sugar, like peanut butter, dried fruit, spaghetti sauce, granola bars, applesauce, chocolate milk, soy milk, and almond milk (look for unsweetened). That's why it's always important to read the ingredient labels!

Don't forget, we are not concerned with calories, but with the quality of the nutrition in the food. The ingredient list will help you tremendously. If you cannot pronounce an ingredient, then it's likely you don't want to serve that food to your family.

Avoid artificial sweeteners, as they can cause stresses and imbalances in susceptible individuals. The three most used and well-known are Splenda (yellow packet), Equal or aspartame (blue packet—most diet soft drinks are made with it), and saccharin (pink packet). Look for words like:

- sugar
- cane sugar
- sucrose
- fructose
- dextrose
- glucose
- maltose
- mannose
- lactose
- sorbitol
- dextrin
- maltodextrin
- monosaccharides
- disaccharides
- agave
- honey
- corn syrup and corn syrup solids

These are all terms for sugar. No matter if it's "organic cane sugar," sugar is sugar. Adding bananas, dates, cinnamon, or unsweetened applesauce to foods is a better approach to sweeten food naturally, as our bodies can better cope with natural rather than artificial foods.

Dispose of processed grains, as many are contaminated with pesticides, chemically adulterated, or have been genetically modified to make them more commercially viable, at the cost of being harder to digest and assimilate. Some common terms for processed grains include: enriched wheat flour, enriched flour, unbleached wheat flour, starch, and modified starch.

If you have junk food at home, chances are your child is going to eat it. Policing the nutritionally poor foods that you've invited into your home is not a sound solution (as we will discuss in the next chapter). It is always better to not have them available at all. If it is in your home, it will end up in your family's bodies.

Junk Food

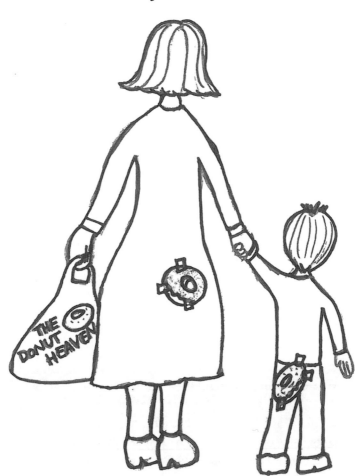

A good rule of thumb is to fill your home with foods that are as natural as possible. In fact, if the foods we're eating are the same types of foods that were around when we were all cave people, then it's natural and is, almost by definition, healthy. If it wasn't around back then, it likely doesn't come from nature and is going to be less healthy for you and your family's bodies.

Our bodies also need certain essential nutrients that junk food and less natural foods don't provide. These nutrients are essential, and because our bodies can't manufacture them from other foods, they have to get them from plants and animals that *can* manufacture them. Some essential nutrients include vitamin C, amino acids, and certain fats.

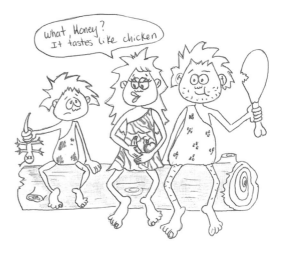

The Problem with Processed Foods

Processed food really starts to sneak in during snacks, so let's start with redefining snack foods.

Snacking is a great and vital part of a healthy diet for children when it involves healthy food. More often than not, however, snacking is an extremely unhealthy habit, where we need little excuse to consume chips, cakes, cookies, and sugary drinks.

A great example of this is Cheetos. The developers of Cheetos have created a snack that is pure sensory pleasure and has what food scientists call "vanishing caloric density." This means that it's consumed quickly, before your brain can register it and send you an "I'm full" signal. This is done on purpose, so you are more likely to overeat its empty calories.[1]

Chips have been put into smaller packages and have even been renamed "baked," so people won't feel so guilty about eating them. Don't be fooled— one-hundred-calorie packages are just another marketing trap. Patients are always so proud to buy them. They are "controlling portions" they say, smiling. But that's part of the problem; we don't want them to control portions! We want children to eat until they are satisfied, really satisfied from being properly nourished. We need to get these chemically laden, poorly nutritious foods out of the house to make room for fruits and vegetables. Fresh fruits and vegetables should be at the top of your list when serving a snack.

Dr. Patricia

Ten years ago, I attended a lecture by a fellow doctor in Texas doing similar work on childhood obesity. He found that obese children were nutritionally deprived. This was a revelation to me: the idea that my patients' constant consumption of nutritionally poor foods may have actually been an attempt to find essential nutrients. This is why I see obesity in homeless children. If you are living on the street in the United States, you are not going to buy broccoli and fresh fruits for your children. Children are going to be fed cookies, pastries, chips, and soda because they won't go bad, they don't need refrigeration, and because when you are just surviving the day-to-day struggle of life on the streets, the last thing you want is an argument with your children about food.

We tell our patients to get rid of all foods the caveman didn't have access to—processed foods, like chips, cereals, most crackers, and hot dogs. Buying cheap, processed foods is a false economy. Whatever money you save buying junk food, you'll end up spending on medical bills, not to mention all the pain and suffering that result from all the bad health that comes from poor eating.

Now that the refrigerator has been purged, the second step is a new shopping list and restocking your home with delicious, nourishing, *real* food.

- **Make a list.** Read on, and we'll tell you what to put on that list. Make sure you do not replenish with the unhealthy food you just got rid of.
- **Don't go grocery shopping when you are hungry.** When your sugar levels are low, you will be craving junk food and will be less likely to make good shopping decisions.
- **Get ready to read.** You are going to have to read labels. Or better yet, pick food without an ingredient list (like fruits, veggies, eggs, chicken, and nuts).

- **Shop the perimeter of the grocery store.** In general, real foods are the ones that require refrigeration or freezing. Typically, a grocery store is set up with the refrigerated areas along the wall. So always start with the perimeter of the store first. That's where you'll find the healthiest, most easily digested foods. You'll also find frozen pizzas, fish fingers, and ice cream, but we're sure you'll know the difference.

Now, let's get started with some specifics, so you know what to shop for.

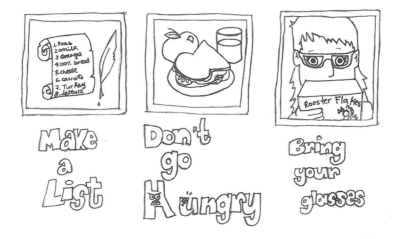

Drinks

First, let's focus on sugary drinks, the usual suspects when it comes to empty calories and unhealthy living. Research has found that consumption of sugar-sweetened drinks is associated with obesity in children.[2] Many of the children who have quickly lost the most weight at Dr. Patricia's clinic have been the ones whose families have gotten rid of sugary drinks and stopped buying them. Examples of sugary drinks: soda pop, sports drinks, fruit juice (even 100 percent fruit juice), chocolate milk, lemonade, punch, many of the commercially available shakes, sweetened coffee drinks, "energy" drinks, and yogurt drinks. Here is a breakdown of sugar content in some commonly consumed kids' drinks:

- Orange juice: 1.5 tablespoons (22.2 grams) in 8 ounces (250 milliliters)
- Apple juice: 1.7 tablespoons (25.1 grams) in 8 ounces
- Mountain Dew: 2.1 tablespoons (31.1 grams) in 8 ounces

- Gatorade: 0.9 tablespoons (13.3 grams) in 8 ounces
- Milk shakes: 3.2 tablespoons (47.3 grams) in 8 ounces
- Chocolate milk: 1.6 tablespoons (23.7 grams) in 8 ounces
- Coke: 1.5 tablespoons (22.2 grams) in 8 ounces

Not only are food portion sizes two to five times bigger than they were in years past, but beverage portions have grown as well. In the mid-1970s, the average sugar-sweetened beverage was 13.6 ounces, but today, kids think nothing of drinking 20 ounces of sugary drinks at a time.[3] On average, Americans consume 100 pounds of sugar and sweeteners each year, or almost 30 teaspoons a day, and nearly half of that comes from soda and fruit drinks.[4] Have you gotten all these usual suspects out of your home yet?

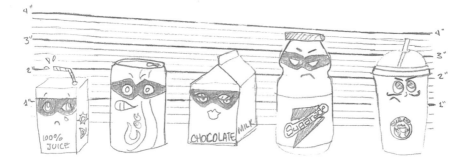

Water, Water, Water

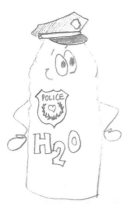

As we start to fill in the basics on your shopping list, don't forget that consuming sugary drinks can lead more easily to dehydration, which can, in turn, stress your body and flip on that FAT switch.

When choosing what drinks to buy, stick to the following question: what did the caveman and cavewoman drink? Answer: water, water, water!

What would happen to fish and plants if we watered them with soda or a sports drink? Why would we give those things to our family, then? In fact, some scientists suspect that, as a whole, we don't drink nearly enough water and that most of us are in a state of chronic dehydration.[5]

We often confuse thirst and hunger; we think that we feel hungry when in reality we're thirsty. The reason for this is that most natural foods——fresh fruit,

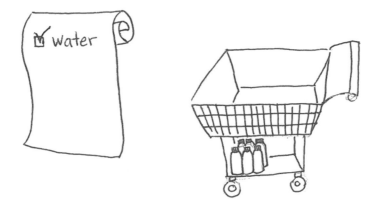

vegetables, meat, eggs, and so on, the type of foods that need refrigeration to stay fresh—are water-rich foods, so when we eat natural foods, we're satisfying hunger and thirst at the same time. This natural signal obviously gets corrupted in a society filled with calorie-dense, but water-poor, foods like white bread, potato chips, and candy bars. The simple way to get around this, when you or your child feels hungry, is to assume that what you're actually feeling is thirst, and drink water. If that doesn't work, and the feeling of hunger is still there, attempt to satiate that hunger with natural, water-rich food, rather than high-calorie, water-poor food.

You do not have to buy bottled water either. You can get a water filter and have an endless supply at home. Ideally, you want water filtered for chlorine, since chlorine can kill friendly bacteria in your gut. A good carbon filter should be fine, but check with your local water distributor if reverse osmosis is necessary to effectively purify your water. Also, if you do buy bottled water, buy bisphenol A (BPA)-free or unde-tected, if possible. BPA is an industrial chemi-cal used to make plastic. You should avoid it. (We will discuss this more in chapter 6).

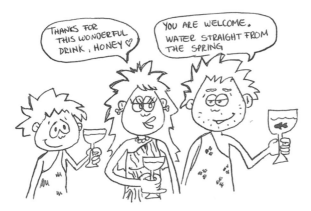

What is the best, most natural drink for babies? Breast milk is best—just a reminder as, obviously, it is not going to be on your shopping list, but it should be on your radar if your child is under one year old or you are planning to have more children. A child's first drink should be breast milk, which is also 80 percent water and is adequate for hydration. In fact, infants should not be given water alone because it can bring down their sodium levels enough to cause seizures.[6] Water from an external source can be introduced at four to six months, as solids are introduced.

Mothers should try to breastfeed for at least the first year of the baby's life. Studies have suggested that breastfeeding is associated with a reduction in the risk of childhood obesity.[7] Breastfeeding protects against disease, food allergies, ear infections, asthma, constipation, and diarrhea. It also improves jaw development, supports immunity, and prevents obesity.[8,9] Breast milk is, naturally, the perfect nutrient for newborns. Remember, an ounce of prevention is worth a pound of cure.

What about Fruit Drinks?

It may seem contrary to some parents, but reducing their children's intake of fruit juice and increasing their intake of whole fruits is a promising strategy for early obesity prevention.[10] Children should eat whole fruits as opposed to drinking fruit juice, even 100 percent juice. Don't believe us? The following is a little story about the Florida orange that illustrates why fruit juice isn't all it's cracked up to be.

The story of how orange juice became a "health drink" says more about the business of factory agriculture than about good nutrition. Orange juice became popular in the twentieth century after Florida found itself plagued with a surplus of oranges they needed to get rid of.[11] Florida growers, in collusion with their state government, marketed orange juice as the latest "health drink," and they were able to successfully sell it as a part of your daily balanced breakfast. Despite its high sugar content and minimal fiber, television shows and commercials still portray healthy people drinking it in the morning. To get even greater market share,

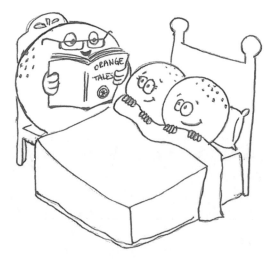

they later introduced a campaign that boasted, "Orange juice. It's not just for breakfast anymore."[12]

When you donate blood, the nurses give you juice and a cookie afterward. Did you ever wonder why? Well, it gets your blood sugar up so fast, you don't feel dizzy. But in normal circumstances, elevating your blood sugar too quickly confuses your body and causes it to overproduce the fat-making hormone, *insulin*. Your body then goes into fat production mode. A short time later, your blood sugar quickly plummets, causing you to feel tired and hungry again. Then you end up eating more junk food and drinking more juice, simply to maintain blood sugar because it is fluctuating so rapidly.

Managing your child's blood sugar is crucial to weight loss, and we'll explore the concept more in coming chapters. But suffice it to say, there is no need to buy juice or other sugary drinks. It is far better to offer your child water and sliced whole fruit than to serve him or her fruit juice.

TASTY TIPS

A few tips if you want to offer some alternative drinks (besides just water) to add variety:

- Decaf herbal teas are fine, as long as they are unsweetened. Mint and chamomile are great examples.
- Slice up fruit, like tangerines or cucumbers, and put it in a pitcher of water. Leave it in the fridge, and the water will absorb the flavor.
- Vegetable shakes or other healthy shakes (look in the recipe section).
- Note: Make sure your plastic bottles and containers are BPA-free.

Fruit

All Whole, Fresh Fruits Are Good

Be prepared to include fresh fruits (and vegetables, for that matter, which we'll cover in the next section) in all meals and snacks. Some may need to be heartier for travel in school lunches or as snacks on the go. Regardless, be liberal with buying and growing and, most importantly, serving fruits.

Fruits are a great source of vitamin C, antioxidants, and other marvelous components that are amazing for your body. For example, whole fruits contain phytochemicals, which protect against cancer and aging, and fiber, which prevents

Bowtie & Grandma

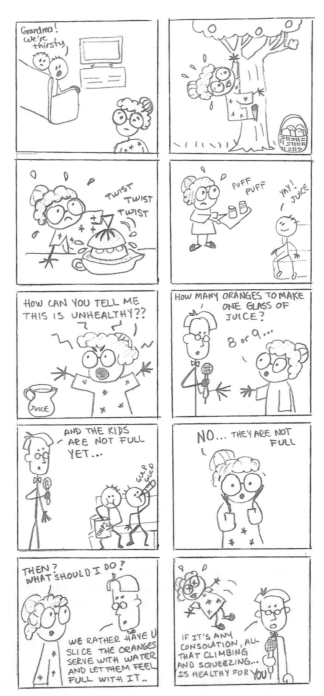

constipation, reduces cholesterol, and helps control weight.[13] There are also anti-oxidants, which are substances found in many foods (especially fruits) that protect your cells against damage, disease, and cancer.[14] Some especially wonderful fruits packed with antioxidants and nutrients include: strawberries, blackberries, blue-berries, papaya, oranges, apples, cherries, pineapple, and apricots.

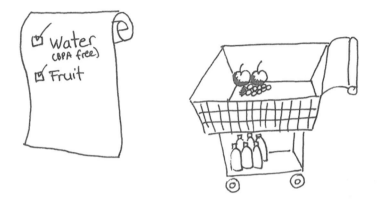

Eating a variety of foods is always the objective, since each food has unique nutrients and qualities. One trick we use, to both add variety to the foods we serve and keep costs down, is to select foods that are in season, which are, conveniently, also usually cheaper and tastier. Check out the Harvest app for your phone at harvest-app.com, which lets you see what's in season in your area and learn how to pick the best produce.

If you can, choose organic fruit. It is a more natural, and therefore, better option, but only if price and budget permits. Organic food is produced on farms that avoid using any fertilizers, pesticides, and additives.[15] A great amount of literature has documented the benefits of eating organically produced fruits and vegetables—these benefits include lower rates of obesity, cardiovascular disease, and cancer. Though this can be controversial, it seems intuitive and logical to strive to offer your family foods that are in their most natural state. But if cost is a factor, don't worry about buying organic fruits, just look to get those that are locally grown, in season, and preferably spray free. *Spray free* means that it's not certified organic, but the producer doesn't spray the food with chemicals. It's often an affordable option to organic.

For foods with thick skins, like pineapple, avacado, or grapefruit, the difference between organic and conventional may not be that great.[16] But for fruits like berries, which are thin skinned and grow low to the ground, it's more important, so you may want to make organic berries a priority on your grocery list. Better yet, if possible, plant some fruit trees or berries in your backyard or on your patio. Kids love gardening. Most children find the whole process of planting a seed, watering it, and watching it grow really exciting. We find that children are much more likely to eat fruits and vegetables when they've participated in the growing process.

Vegetables

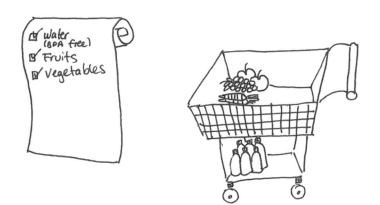

Everyone knows they are good for you, but nobody seems to want to eat them.

Vegetables contain a host of good nutrients for your body. Some examples of vegetables to include in your family's diet are: kale, watercress, spinach, broccoli rabe (a stronger-tasting version of conventional broccoli), napa cabbage (also known as Chinese cabbage), Brussels sprouts, and arugula (also known as rocket or rocket lettuce). Live greens, such as sprouts, are an especially great way to go!

If your kids are willing to drink vegetable juice, then we suggest that you go for it, but don't force it. Freshly squeezed vegetable juice is different than fruit juice because it doesn't contain as much sugar.

So how do you get your kids, and the rest of your family, to eat more vegetables? Be persistant and start with the basics: BSE.

> B: Buy them
> S: Serve them
> E: Eat them yourself

Remember, out of sight, out of mind. So put vegetables in sight and in mind, and eventually the vegetables will be in your families' tummies too!

Top Ten Tips to Get Your Kids to Eat Vegetables

All meals and snacks should include fresh fruits or vegetables. There are many strategies for getting your child to eat vegetables:

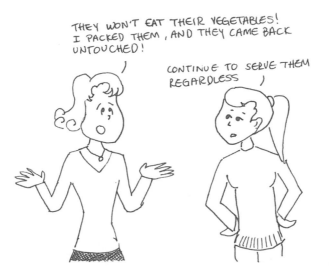

1. **Serve them often.** There's something called the rule of fifteen.[17,18] Children need to be offered bitter foods, like vegetables, fifteen (or up to twenty-eight) times before you know if they'll like them. We saw a demonstration of a cute nine-month-old in a high chair being fed green beans. On day one researchers fed him green beans with a spoon, and he promptly pushed them away. No big deal. These researchers knew they were going to try them again. Day two was the same result, all the way to day twenty-seven. Then on day twenty-eight, with the same baby, the same researcher, and the same spoon, the baby ate the green beans and opened his mouth for more. Houston, we have liftoff!

    Another good strategy is to serve a salad with every meal. Get your kids used to the fact that every good meal includes a salad. Jon recalls a story he heard from one friend in which her six-year-old daughter, when served a dinner without a salad, remarked, "Mommy, where's the salad?" If you consistently serve salad, your child will come to expect the salad and even—believe it or not—eventually look forward to it.

Heather, one of the nutritional coaches on the Gabriel Method team, tells all her clients to serve their food "on top of a salad." This is grat advice because, ideally, a salad should take up the entire plate and not just the side. That's exactly the way Jon eats most of his meals. It's usually one huge salad with lots of animal protein and healthy dressing.

Remember to try lots of different type of lettuces and combinations of vegetables in your salad. Try different sprouts, like sunflower, lentil, and chickpea sprouts. Kids often love sprouts, and they're full of nutrients, affordable, and usually organic. They're also very easy to grow at home. Remember to add salad and sprouts to sandwiches, wraps, tacos, and burritos too.

2. **Avoid labeling your kids with their food preferences.** Most of us offer green beans to our child a couple of times and then turn to our spouse and say, "The kid doesn't like green beans," and then we stop serving them. This attitude of giving up too soon defeats vegetable eating in two ways: first, you stop serving them, and second, you label your child as a "green-bean hater." We hear people labeling their children with their food preferences all the time. "He likes this." "She's a good eater." "He eats portions that are too big." "She hates vegetables." Unfortunately, labeling is just creating self-fulfilling prophecies that make things worse.[19]

Prophecy Fulfilled

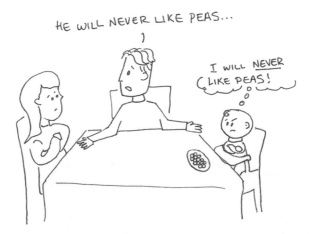

3. **Start with the vegetables that you know your child likes and build from there.** If they like salads, try different green leaves or radishes or other

vegetables, and build as you go. If they like carrots, then serve carrots, but add some other vegetables on the side.

4. **Avoid coaxing or bribing.** Refrain from making comments designed to coax your child into eating vegetables. "I made these tomatoes especially for you." "Just try it." "You need to try one bite." Believe us when we tell you that if there were a specific tag line you could just say that would magically get children to eat vegetables immediately, we'd tattoo it onto our own forearms and onto the forearms of every parent, and we would read it aloud at every meal and snack. But the fact is studies show that if you coax children to eat a food, even if they do try it, the next time they are offered that food, they are less likely to eat it.[20] Bribing is just as counterproductive as coaxing, so refrain from bribing at the table.[21] It's a slippery slope, teaming with unhealthy food relationship issues. So avoid statements like, "If you finish your vegetables, you can have dessert."

5. **Avoid bullying and threatening.** Refrain from statements like, "You will be grounded because you didn't eat your Brussels sprouts." Bullying doesn't work and is yet another tactic that sets up a dysfunctional relationship with food.

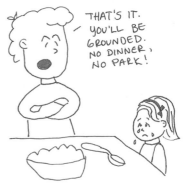

6. **Eat vegetables yourself.** Back to BSE. Buy them, serve them, and *eat* them yourself. Set an example, and your kids will do as you do. Studies show that if Mom eats vegetables, the child is more likely to eat them.[22] We figure that this is true for fathers too. Also, even in utero or when nursing, children develop a taste for vegetables more when their mothers are eating them.[23]

7. **Get children involved with gardening and growing their own vegetables, or take them to visit a farm.** Studies have found that gardening with children has positive effects, including improved attitudes toward vegetables, recognition of vegetables, and vegetable consumption.[24,25]

8. **Let them play with their food.** If it's appropriate to your child's age or level of development, then let them play with their food. Many of us were taught that playing with food was a no-no, but for many children, playing with their food is a healthy way for them to experience different types

of foods, especially if they are resistant to trying new foods.[26] In our Stone Soup program, the classes that Dr. Patricia's team runs for pre-schoolers, we let children explore their food, allowing them to play

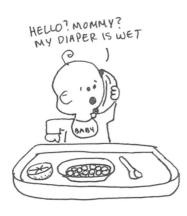

with fresh vegetables and even letting the children paint with them. By the same token, let younger children get messy with their food. Schedule baths after meals or use bibs to avoid huge messes, but let them get their hands dirty and explore their food when they are young.

9. **Get children involved in preparing vegetables.** When Dr. Patricia's daughter was about four, they were in the grocery store when a woman offering store samples asked the little girl, "Would you like to try some ranch dressing? Kids love it." Dr. Patricia cringed at the coaxing, but let it go. Her daughter said, "No, thank you, but that is my favorite lettuce. Can I have some without dressing?" Now, this child (an obvious outlier to the rule of fifteen), had been offered salad for three years or more and, to her mother's frustration, had only tried it one time. The lettuce she was pointing to was butter lettuce, one of the types they regularly bought. She took the paper cup from the lady and started munching on the lettuce in the store like it was a cookie. Dr. Patricia was shocked, but kept it inside as the wheels in her head churned. She then asked her daughter, "Would you like to get your own lettuce to take home to help me make a rainbow salad?" "Sure, Mom," she said.

She was into rainbows at the time, so they picked different fruits and vegetables for each color in the rainbow. But there was a catch: "But Mom, please, no dressing." Who knew that the dressing, the least nutritious part of the salad, had been the barrier all along? Dr. Patricia knew that had she made a comment in those previous three years that her daughter didn't like salads, the situation would never have worked out the way it did. Her daughter would have bought into the "reality" that "she doesn't like salads" if Dr. Patricia had pointed it out and repeated it often enough. But salads were never the problem, and they still make rainbow salads to this day.

10. **Turn it into arts and crafts.** Children love to use food to make art projects, and when they do, they're much more likely to eat the food afterward. Jon's family often makes a pizza omelet, using a thin, flat-egg omelet for the base, instead of pizza dough. They make the omelet and put it on a plate with lots of colorful veggies to choose from, then let the kids decorate the omelet. They make smiley faces with peppers and olives. They use mushrooms to make ears and noses, sprouts to make facial hair, and corn for teeth. The kids love getting involved this way and sometimes even have competitions for the best faces.

Bonus tip: Take a deep breath. The more stressed out you feel about your child not eating vegetables, the more stressed out your child will feel as well. Give yourself a pat on the back from us if you serve vegetables often. Don't base your success with vegetables on whether your child eats them or how much they eat, which we will go into in more depth when we discuss the psychology of feeding children in the next chapter. Stick to your new mantra: BSE. *Buy* them, *serve* them, and *eat* them yourself. Never make a child eat his or her vegetables. Why? Because it doesn't work, and it is counterproductive in establishing a healthy, psychologically sound way of feeding children.

Protein

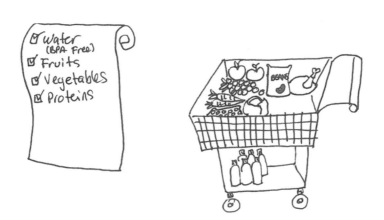

Protein can come from plants or animals and should be on everyone's grocery list. Proteins in food are made from amino acids, which are needed to build the proteins necessary for our bodies. We can make twelve of these amino acids ourselves, but there are eight that we need to obtain from the foods we eat. Proteins from animals include: beef, chicken, turkey, fish, eggs, pork, and so on. Fish, like salmon, are rich in omega-3 fatty acids, which, if consumed regularly (at least once a week), have been shown to decrease the risk of heart attack.[27]

Some plant proteins that you might not have on your radar are: nuts, nut butters, and seeds. When you shop for them, make sure there are no added sugars, oils, or other chemicals. Raw and in the

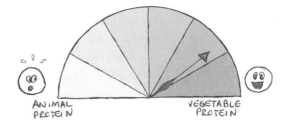

ANIMAL PROTEIN   VEGETABLE PROTEIN

shell is the most healthy form of nut (which is more like how a caveperson would have eaten them), but be careful with children under four, as they can choke on nuts and seeds. As long as there are no allergies, it's better to give nut butters and wait until they are older for the other forms of nuts and seeds.

The more nourished your body, the more satisfied you feel after eating, so the end result is that you eat less. Natural seeds and nuts, for example, are concentrated foods rich in vitamins, minerals, proteins, and good oils. Experience tells you that you don't need much of them to feel full.

**FOODS TO AVOID FEEDING CHILDREN
UNDER THE AGE OF FOUR**

According to the American Academy of Pediatrics, because of the potential choking risk for children under four years of age, you should avoid feeding them the following:

- No hard, smooth foods that have to be chewed with a grinding motion. This includes peanuts and raw vegetables.
- No round, firm foods, like carrots, unless they are chopped completely, like carrot sticks.
- No gum, grapes, or popcorn.

One important point: do not buy nuts roasted in vegetable oil, as this type of oil can cause inflammation and lead to weight gain. It's not that oil is bad for you. Some oils are essential and extremely beneficial. It's just that the type of oil matters (as we'll talk about in a minute). As we said before, raw is ideal, but even better than raw is *activated*. That's when the nut is soaked overnight and slightly sprouted. This process of activating nuts breaks down the outer wall of the nut and makes the nutrients more available and easier to digest. But if not raw or activated, then dry-roasted is best. But please read the label and make sure there's no vegetable oil, sugar, or artificial flavorings in either the dry-roasted or the raw nuts.

The best quality of animal foods comes from animals that eat the food found in nature. Take great care when selecting animal proteins like steak, chicken, turkey, eggs, pork, fish, and so on.

For example, wild fish is better than farm-raised fish; free-range chickens and eggs are better than their factory-farmed counterparts; and grass-fed beef is healthier than grain-fed beef. The difference in nutrition between naturally

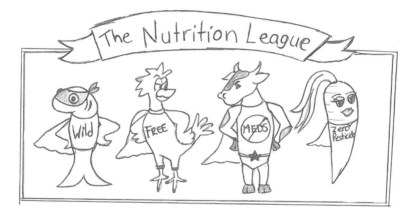

fed animals and those that are not naturally fed can be incredible. Beef from grass-fed cattle is much more nutritionally beneficial, containing lower levels of unhealthy fats and cholesterol and higher levels of omega-3 fatty acids and vitamins A and E.[28]

Although it can be more expensive, when you're able to and when you have the choice, naturally fed meat is a better route. And don't forget, you might be more satisfied and eat less since it is higher in nutrition, which would help your pocketbook. Also, when you take these fabulous proteins home, grill, bake, or broil them, but please avoid frying them.

Avoid processed meats, such as sausage, bologna, pepperoni, and hot dogs. Processed meat can be defined as any meat preserved by smoking, curing, or salting. These foods have excessive chemicals, sugars, and salts and are associated with increased risk of diabetes, stroke, and coronary heart disease.[29]

Whole Grains

This is a controversial food and with good reason! It seems like grain products have been tampered with more than any other food group. Ultimately, these foods were not the foods that cavemen and hunter-gatherers had on their dinner plates. Bread, rice, crackers, cereals, corn chips, oatmeal, pasta, and tortillas—they are all highly susceptible to tampering, and you bet the food industry has had a field day tinkering with them. Kellogg's cereal was originally supposed to be a health food, but all that changed when one brother bought out the other and discarded the health food concept, gearing his efforts toward marketing the brand and increasing advertising.[30] And it worked.

Many of our most common and most unhealthy meals and snacks are made up largely of processed grains. Processed grains are the worst of all because they have lost 80 to 90 percent of their nutrients, including fiber, vitamins, minerals, and phytochemicals. Compared to whole grains, they contribute to higher blood-sugar spikes, which result in higher insulin spikes.

Processed grains include foods like: white bread, "wheat" bread, white rice, white noodles, white flour tortillas, white crackers, most breakfast cereals, wheat flour, enriched wheat flour, unbleached wheat flour, starch, and modified starch. Also, don't be fooled by labels like "multigrain." Rather, look for a label that says "100 percent whole grain"—though we also find that even whole grain products are often laden with added sugar, particularly breakfast cereals.

Bread, whether whole grain or not, usually has some added sugar as well. Read the ingredient list. The best breads to choose have a short list of ingredients, the grains will have the word "whole" in front of them, and there won't be any added sugars. Other key words to watch out for are "stoneground" and "sprouted." Stoneground, whole-grain flours and sprouted whole grains have a larger particle size than most other flours, and are known for lower insulin spikes,[31] increased nutrient retention, and greater bulking effect for regularity and intestinal health.[32]

Fats

Not all fats are the same. Not all fats are equal. At a molecular level, fatty acids look like strings, and it's the shape of the strings that determines how the fat behaves. We usually refer to fats that are solid at room temperature as *fats* and those that are liquid at room temperature as *oils*.

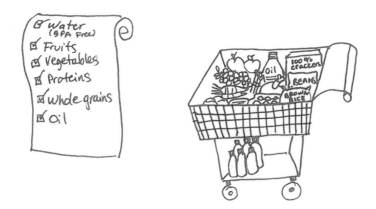

- Some fat strings are straight. These are the saturated fats, and they're more likely to be solid at room temperature.
- Some fat strings have a single bend or kink in them. These are the monounsaturated fats, and they're more likely to be liquid at room temperature.
- Some fat strings have more than one kink in them. These are the polyunsaturated fats, and they're liquid at room temperature.
- In nature, many of the fats that come from unprocessed food are the monounsaturated and polyunsaturated types, but modern industrial processing tends to change the nature of these fats, corrupting them into the straight-lined, saturated fats.

Getting Kinky with Fats

Omega-3 fatty acids are a particularly good type of fat. Structurally, they have a kink in just the right place and in just the right way to reduce inflammation in the body. Inflammation is a phenomenon that is largely observed in, and linked to, obesity.[33] In a natural diet, there's a one-to-one ratio of omega-3s to omega-6s, another group of good fats. Again, unfortunately, modern growing and processing methods tamper with this ratio, and this triggers an inflammatory response in the human body.

Omega-3 fatty acids can help lower cholesterol, reduce inflammation in the body, and reduce the risk of heart disease, and nutritionists recommend consuming them twice a week.[34,35,36]

Mass food producers and marketers don't like omega-3s because they're a lot more fragile than saturated fats. Omega-3s don't like heat, and they don't like light. As a result, the fat sources that are rich in omega-3s, like flaxseed, chia-seed, and hempseed oil, aren't the best fats to cook with, and you're better off using them in salad dressings. Another great way to get omega-3s in your diet is to sprinkle chia seeds or ground flaxseeds on cold food or into shakes.

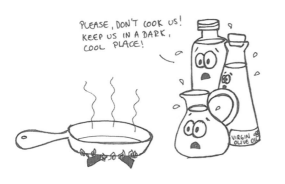

For cooking, the best oils are cold-pressed and resistant to burning. If an oil burns at too low a temperature, like canola oil (which is a processed oil), it becomes denatured and less healthy.

The best oils for frying are: ghee (clarified butter), cold-pressed coconut, cold-pressed grape-seed, cold-pressed rice-bran, or cold-pressed avocado oil. If you don't have access to these, at least see if you can get your hands on some cold-pressed olive oil, also known as extra-virgin olive oil.

As Natural as Possible

Double-check your shopping cart. Ask yourself, is everything as natural as possible? This means, for the most part, ignoring most of what you'll find in the center aisles of the supermarket and sticking to the perimeter, where you find the fresh fruits and vegetables and refrigerated meats and eggs. It means avoiding sugary drinks, especially soda pop with its artificial colorants (even if the label says "natural colors") and artificial sweeteners, like aspartame. It means, when possible, avoiding grain-fed meats riddled with growth hormones and antibiotics. As raw, natural, and unprocessed as possible is the general rule to follow to get the most nutrition out of food.

Miscellaneous Foods That Are Good for Digestion

Naturally fermented live foods, such as miso (fermented soybean paste), tempeh (cultured soybeans), tamari (wheat-free soy sauce), sauerkraut (German-style fermented cabbage), kim chee (Korean-style cabbage or other vegetables fermented in chili), nutritional yeast (also known as "brewer's yeast"), yogurt, and kefir are full of friendly bacteria and enzymes that help digestion. Another great source of friendly gut bacteria is probiotics. You can take probiotics as tablets, but they're also available as powders. You can add the probiotic powder to smoothies.

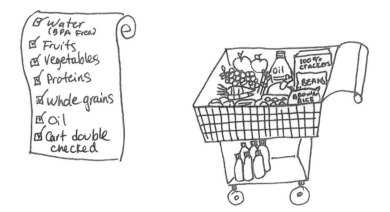

More and more studies are being published that demonstrate the importance of friendly bacteria in health and weight loss. A particularly interesting study involved twins, one thin and the other overweight. The researchers took samples of the intestinal bacteria from the overweight twin and injected it into the intestines of mice, and amazingly the mice gained weight. They repeated the experiment with the bacteria from the thin twin, and the mice with this bacteria didn't gain any weight. What's more, when they injected the bacteria of the thin twin into the mice that had just gained weight, they actually lost weight.[37]

While we do not fully understand the role of friendly bacteria in health and weight loss, it is becoming increasingly clear that a healthy gut equals a healthy body.

Grocery Shopping Tips

- Plan to make one shopping trip per week to get the majority of what you need. Then, plan for a second trip in the middle of the week to restock fresh foods.
- If possible, have a list in hand when you go to the grocery store. Review the grocery ads, and write your list according to what is on sale. Whatever is in season is typically on sale, which means you are getting a deal on the food at a time when it tastes the best.
- Keep your list in a handy spot so that you can add to it during the week. Make a note to restock any essential items.
- Plan to use specific ingredients in multiple ways throughout the week. For example, if broccoli is a really good price, plan to use it in stir-fry, soup, and as a side dish.
- If your children go to the store with you, and they are old enough to be away from you for a few minutes, give them a specific item to find in the store. This will give them a sense of accomplishment and help them learn what types of foods are healthy.
- Encourage your children to explore the produce section. Ask them to pick out a fruit or vegetable that they have never tasted before or to find a fruit or vegetable that is a certain color.
- The grocery store is filled with temptations for all of us. Be prepared to give a firm no when your child requests junk food.
- Wash fruits and vegetables when you get home. Package them up for easy grab-and-go snacks, or leave them easily visible in the refrigerator. Refill your fruit bowl, and leave it out where it is easily accessible and attractive. Showcase the beautiful in-season fruits and vegetables! Don't ever underestimate the additional attraction of fruits and vegetables that have been cut and served.

Go to TheGabrielMethod.com/FitKids and DrRibasHealthClub.org /FitKids for lots of simple, yummy recipe ideas.

Additional Information about Ingredients to Avoid

Avoid monosodium glutamate (MSG). This flavor enhancer, found in most packaged snack foods and canned goods, has been linked to obesity. In research published in the *American Journal of Clinical Nutrition* in June 2011, nutrition expert Ka He and his colleagues found that, "Men and women who ate the most MSG (a median of 5 grams a day) were about 30 percent more likely to become overweight by the end of the study than those who ate the least amount of the flavoring (less than a half of a gram a day) . . . After excluding people who were overweight at the start of the study, the risk rose to 33 percent."[38]

Here's a little-known fact outside of research laboratories: when scientists, for whatever reason, need to study fat mice or rats, they make them gain weight by deliberately feeding them MSG. There's even a specific name for them too: *MSG obesity-induced mice.* In other words, in scientific circles the fact that MSG causes obesity is taken for granted.

Avoid aspartame, the current artificial sweetener of choice for many so-called diet drinks. Artificial sweeteners in general have had a checkered history. Lead acetate, a sweetener used in ancient Rome, was eventually found to be highly toxic. Then there's cyclamate. The US Food and Drug Administration banned cyclamate in 1970 after it was found to cause bladder cancer in lab rats, but it's still used in many parts of the world, including Europe.

Avoid saccharin. Invented in 1879, it is permitted in the United States but restricted elsewhere and banned in many other countries. Not that natural sugar is all that great either.

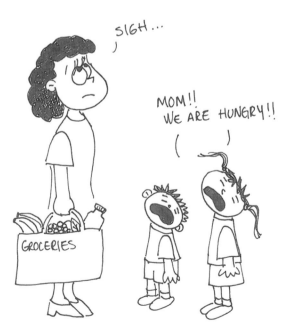

The idea of sugar as sweet poison has been explored extensively, and more and more people are beginning to take notice of just how bad too much sugar—the king of empty carbs—can be for the body. However, a study conducted by Purdue University in 2008 showed that "rats fed yogurt sweetened with sugar did not eat as much as the rats fed artificially sweetened yogurt. The premise is that eating real sugar sets off a response that lets the body know that real calories are being consumed. In turn, the rat feels satisfied after eating."[39]

What's true for mice and rats might not be true for humans, but we need to consider the possibility that artificial sweeteners may bypass the body's natural warning system for calorie consumption, thus making us want to consume more food than is necessary. This brings us back to aspartame, a close chemical relative to aspartic acid, which is actually completely natural and one of the most common amino acids. Aspartame itself, however, often sold under the brand name NutraSweet, is the subject of continuing controversy, with many authorities considering it harmless and others linking it to obesity.[40]

In short, we'd generally advise against artificial sweeteners. Instead, we use apples, dates, bananas, cinnamon, and unsweetened applesauce to naturally sweeten food. Based on our knowledge today, coconut palm sugar, xylitol, and stevia are all natural substances which, when used in the right proportions, provide sweetness without causing the blood-sugar spikes of table sugar or the toxicity of artificial sweeteners.

So now you've finished your grocery shopping, and you've brought all your food home. Now, what do you do?

4

The Psychology of Feeding Children

What was the dynamic at the dinner table when you were growing up? Did you have to clean your plate? Did you have to finish your food because "people were starving in other countries?" Did you have to eat your vegetables to get dessert? Were you considered "good" or "bad" depending on what or how much you ate? Were you told which foods you could have seconds of and which you couldn't? Have you perpetuated any of these behaviors in your own home now?

These are all dysfunctional scenarios that lead to unhealthy relationships with food. Understanding the psychology of feeding your child is one of the best tools you can use to help your child let go of the hoarding and food scarcity mentality that can lead to overeating.

The Psychology of Feeding

The psychology of feeding your child is essential to establishing a healthy feeding dynamic with your child—heck, with your whole family for that matter. Inspired by Ellyn Satter's brilliant writings on the "Division of Responsibility in Feeding,"[1] we've laid out some important ground rules that you can follow when feeding your child.

To begin:

- Know your role in the feeding relationship.
- You cannot and do not want to cross the line.

- Stick to your role, and know that it is all that you can control.
- Enjoy meals with your family.

Bowtie & the Frazzled Mom

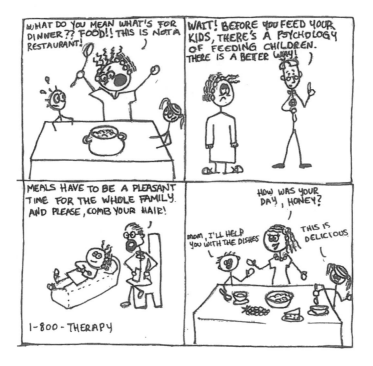

Your child is responsible for whether or not to eat the choices of food you offer, as well as how much of it he or she eats, but what about the parents' role? Here are five tips for making mealtimes more enjoyable:

1. **You are in charge of what to serve.** You just cleaned out the cupboards. You went shopping and restocked them with healthy food. No matter what you serve now, it should all have loads of nutrition, and you ought to feel good about that. You get a star from us. You filled your house with healthy food, and you are serving that healthy food. So you know your family will be eating nutritious food, and that is an amazing accomplishment. Well done!

2. **You are in charge of when to serve the food.** Generally, feed children every two to three hours, serving three meals and two to three snacks a

day. We recommend serving breakfast within a half hour of waking up. Then offer food about every two to three hours after that. This works even when children are in school or on the go. So, breakfast, snack, lunch, snack, dinner, and optional snack (don't forget snacks start with fresh fruit and vegetables). Don't ask them if they're hungry. Just serve it. They will eat if they are hungry, as long as the psychology is sound. For children at school, be sure to pack a snack with their lunch and another for after school or on the go, if necessary.

3. **You are in charge of setting the tone for meals and snacks.** Turn off all electronics, especially the television. Children who are distracted by television at meals are less likely to be in tune with when their tummies are hungry or full. Music may actually add to your ambiance, so you can use it if you want. But cell phones, newspapers, television, toys, and videogames should not be allowed at the table.

Most importantly, keep your stresses and the daily grind away from meals and keep them out of mealtime dynamics. You worked all day—you may have shopped, cooked, cleaned, put out fires, and now you have to set the table. Take a deep breath. This is your precious time with the people you love most in your life. Leave your day's stress behind you. Protect this time with your loved ones and eliminate negativity from the crazy world we live in. This is not the time to pick a fight with your spouse or bring up flammable topics. Nourish your family with love at the table. We will follow up on the dos and don'ts of what to say in the next section. For now, bring your heart to the table and leave your sword at the door.

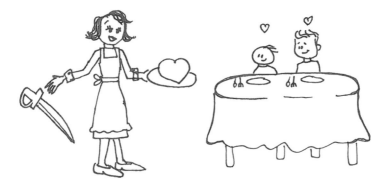

4. **Make sure the whole family comes together.** Pick mealtimes when the most family members can participate. Most of us have busy schedules.

Your children should not be up in their room, and neither should a parent or grandfather, when the family is having a meal. They don't have to eat, but they should join the family at the table. This time should be the pinnacle of your relationship with your family, and it should help strengthen the bond and communication between family members. Children who have regular family meals do better with respect to avoiding drugs, alcohol, and early sexual behavior. Family meals in a child's life translate into more positive outcomes than do sports, tutors, church, and music lessons.[2]

5. **Make it fun.** You don't have to be Martha Stewart or Valerie Rice to integrate some creativity and fun into meals. For example, choosing napkins that reflect a holiday, cooking foods that reflect the season, lighting a candle, or setting decorations on the table. You or your kids can gather flowers from the garden, pinecones, leaves, or add figurines for décor. Put a board game or cards near the table to enjoy after the meal. You can even put a tablecloth outside or place a picnic blanket on the floor in the family room in front of the fire, which can make a regular meal feel much more special, inviting, and fun!

It is critical for children to enjoy meals with their family. If this mealtime environment isn't established, children won't have it as part of their foundation. Then, as they get older, they will go out or to friends' homes for meals. A healthy mealtime environment in your home, however, is likely to make their friends want to come to your house to have meals. Start now, no matter how old your kids are. Begin to enjoy meals together today.

If left to his or her own devices, when a child is hungry, he or she will eat. When children are not hungry, they won't want to eat and no amount of threatening and cajoling will have any effect. It's better to simply let children experience the natural consequences of hunger so that they maintain their natural feeding pattern. The rule should be that everyone must come to the table, but *if* or *how much* they eat is up to the individual (yes, that means the child can decide if and how much he or she is going to eat).

This concept is not new; it was illustrated in the 1904 book *The Secret Garden*. The book's heroine is a young girl, spoiled by nannies. These nannies would make multiple meals to please her, but to no avail. Her parents both subsequently die of cholera, and the orphaned child goes to live with her uncle in the United Kingdom. Her uncle keeps his distance, so the housekeeper becomes her caretaker. The housekeeper is the oldest child of a large, poor family, so though cheerful, she isn't the type to put up with any rubbish from anybody. She makes breakfast the first day, but the girl refuses it and wants something else. The housekeeper chuckles and, with a smile, says that she'll eat when she's hungry. No drama. No judgment. So the girl goes without breakfast and goes outside to play, gets some sun on her cheeks, and works up an appetite. The next day, she eats the porridge that the housekeeper serves.

We realize that simply letting go and not insisting that your kids eat their Brussels sprouts might run counter to your cultural biases or your instinct that says that if they don't eat, they'll suffer some horrible fate. The fact is that if you establish normal feeding patterns and eliminate the availability of junk foods in the house, your children's bodies will know better at a moment-by-moment level what they need even more than you do.

Ultimately, this is the answer to getting them to eat what you want them to eat. It's about letting go, but letting go after you've created a nonthreatening environment in which healthy choices are abundant and available. Unrestricted eating is the basis for a healthy relationship with food. As we keep reiterating, restriction (portion control) leads to food insecurity where kids may:

- Be worried that they'll be hungry and won't get enough food
- Binge, hoard, or hide food
- Feel guilty when they do eat

Aren't there enough worries in their lives? We need to stay away from all that negativity. Unrestricted eating does not mean that you let your kids eat whatever they want. Remember, you are in charge of what food is in the house. It means that you make great, healthy, tasty foods available as appealing options, and then you let them self-regulate by letting them decide how much of those great options to eat without restriction, guilt, pressure, or conditions. Children's metabolic needs change from day to day and over time. They could be in a normal growth spurt or more active than usual, or perhaps less active than usual. They could be sick or constipated. They will adjust their portions naturally to compensate. Do not interfere with the natural cues that are affecting their appetite throughout the day and from day-to-day.

You don't want your child to eat in order to please you. Neither do you want to force your child to eat something that she'll rebel against. You want your child to learn a lifelong skill of eating to satisfaction and listening to her tummy to know when to eat and when to stop. Self-regulation is the key. It is a skill that will promote a healthy body for life.

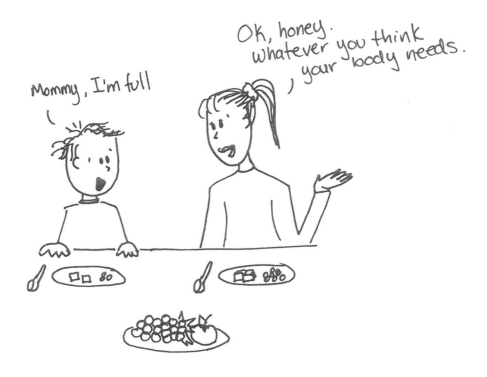

Table Talk

Now that you have learned everyone's job in the feeding relationship, let's work on what to say and not say at the table, which will help set the tone at mealtimes.

You want to engage in upbeat, non-food-related conversation with your family at the dinner table. For example, discuss things that happened throughout the day or over the weekend that the child or family enjoyed, sharing experiences and stories. Expressing gratitude, finding alternative ways to view situations, acting kindly toward others, and giving constructive praise have all been linked to long-term improvements in emotional and physical health and to a decline in depression symptoms.[3] So let your table talk be filled with these messages.

Praise the children's appropriate behavior, describe and reflect on their actions, and express gratitude. For example, "Thank you for helping push your sister's chair in," or "I like the way you were very polite to the teller when we went to the bank today." Kids get bombarded with questions from adults all day long. "How old are you?" "What's your name?" "What's two plus two?" They can shut down. Have you noticed when you ask a teenager how his day was he says, "Fine"? Not very forthcoming with the details, right?

Instead, work on asking open-ended questions and make statements of interest, such as "I would love to hear how ballet class went today," or "Your school project on American heroes sounds cool." This not only encourages the parent to know more about the child's schedule, but it also increases the child's self-esteem and sense of importance. It is important that the praise and reflections are in relation to positive behaviors, not in relation to food choices. This works to take focus off of the food and to establish positive bonding at mealtimes. For example, you would never want to say, "Great job eating your green beans."

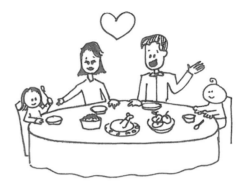

Make sharing fun by going around the table discussing highs and lows of the day or using cards, books, pictures, or random words taken from a dictionary as conversation starters.

WHAT YOU *SHOULD NOT DO* AT THE TABLE:

- Bring the stress from your daily grind
- Limit portions
- Bribe
- Reward with food
- Label your child's food preferences
- Coax your child to eat more or less
- Bully or punish your child to get him to eat more or less
- Force feed your child, no matter how much you want to

WHAT YOU *SHOULD DO* AT THE TABLE:

- Fill your family with love at the table
- Catch your children being good
- Describe good things your children did that day
- Go around the table and share highs and lows of the day

What Not to Say *at the Table:*

- **Portion control:** "Have more of this," or "Don't have so much of that."
- **Artificial or phony comments:** "Yum! These Brussels sprouts are so good!" Don't try to make one food sound more appetizing than another. If it is a sincere comment about the food, it is reasonable.

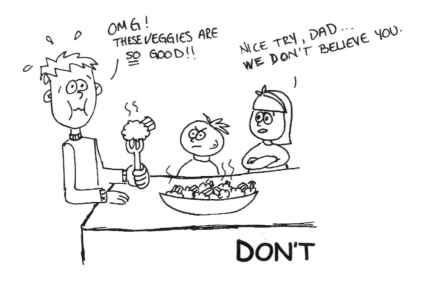

- **Bribing and coaxing:** As in using food as a tool of negotiation. This interrupts the child's intuition and satiety cues, and places negative association upon food. "If you eat your green beans, you can have dessert." You should also aim to stop using food, especially junk food, as a bribe or a reward. This sets up a pattern in which kids associate "being good" with eating badly. In the words of one mother: "[bribing with food] . . . It not only sets up bad eating habits, but it teaches children how to be manipulative."[4] This makes the dessert or unhealthy food become the reward and makes healthy foods seem less appetizing.

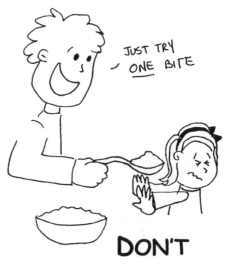

- **Pressuring:** Trying to pressure the child into eating certain foods or behaving a certain way is also not a good idea: "Mmm this broccoli tastes so good," or "Just try one bite. Just one more bite." By trying to pressure your child into eating certain foods, even if she eats it in the moment, she will be less likely to eat it in the future.[5]

- **Rewarding with food:** "If you get good grades, I will take you out for ice cream." There are always other ways to encourage and reward good behavior, like helping kids with a project or doing something fun. You might find that children actually prefer spending quality time with you over eating a candy bar. Reward them with your time and activities, such as books, roller-skating, shooting baskets, and so on, but not with food.

- **Emotional attachment:** Avoid establishing emotional associations with food by using food to comfort or console your child. A study found that, "Parents who use food to satisfy their children's emotional needs or to promote good behavior in their children may promote weight gain by interfering with their children's ability to regulate their own food intake."[6] Once again, give your time or praise instead of food.

- **Labeling:** Defining preferences by telling a child what foods they like or dislike. This suggests to a child that food preferences are rigid and unchanging and hinders their development of a balanced, variable diet.

- **Claiming certain foods are "good" or "bad":** This creates confusion and the idea of forbidden foods. Making statements like "Johnny hates tomatoes" will make the child think he doesn't like something, and he will be much less likely to try it in the future. Making a big fuss if he eats something previously ignored will only make him feel that he's getting unwanted attention.

- **Force-feeding:** Step away from the spoon. Force-feeding is never a good idea because it interrupts the pattern of natural hunger signals. Avoid saying the old classic, "You have to clean your plate."

- **Body shaming:** You can't get kids to eat what you want them to eat by criticizing their bodies. The paradox is that you're much more likely to be able to solve your child's obesity problem if you minimize attention to their body altogether, or to anyone else's body for that matter. So don't refer to yourself, friends, colleagues, relatives, or pop stars by derogatory names for being overweight (fat, fatso, tubby, lard bucket, or any number of other insults), especially if your child is currently overweight. You can't shame someone into thinness.

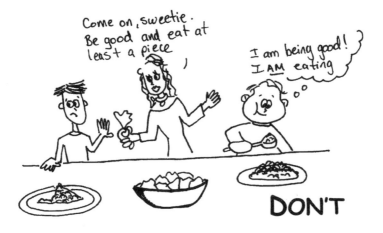

We've said it before, but it's worth repeating: if there is junk food in the house, it will be eaten. The simplest way around this is to stop buying it and putting it there in the first place. And if it is there, either throw it out or give it away. If it's not there in the first place, then nobody's going to be tempted, and nobody's going to have to practice self-discipline to stay away from it. If it's not there, no one has to deny themselves and create the hoarding mentality that contributes to weight gain.

Policing food is not the answer. Everyone in the house should be eating the same way (mom, dad, and kids), and no one should be singled out and put on a diet. Again, the foods we are recommending are the foods that everyone, of

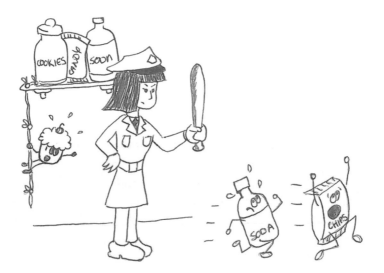

any size and age, should eat. Keeping sweets in the fridge for one kid but not another, hiding leftover Halloween candy, or locking up sweets are all bad ideas.

Dr. Patricia's team uses the same principles to help children who are underweight or who are failing to gain weight. Offering optimum nutrition is ingrained in the principles of healthy eating and apply to everyone. Even if your kids are older, and you have less control than you once had, you can still make a difference now. Don't punish yourself; don't feel that you've missed the boat. Do what you can, set boundaries, and take control of the environment today. First off, relax a little. Start by filling the house with healthy food and making meals a positive experience for yourself and your family. Your actions will speak a million times louder than your words. Make the changes quietly without a big announcement.

TIPS FOR MAKING MEALTIMES MORE PLEASANT:

- Turn off the television.
- Sit down together as a family.
- Offer a variety of healthy foods.
- Love your children at the table.
- Follow the psychology of feeding.

We need to make mealtimes fun.
We need to stop forcing our children to eat or not to eat.
We need to quit controlling portions.
We need to stop putting our children on diets or telling them they need to be on one.

One easy way to get your kids healthier is to help them feel empowered about food. Cook with them! Help them make their own healthy salads or snacks, adding fun elements like smiley faces. Get them engaged with food so that it becomes a friend and not an intimidating enemy. If you can associate healthy food with fun, then the battle is half-won. You can make kids' natural tendency to play with food work to everyone's advantage.

If you have the space and time, growing your own food is a fabulous way to get kids engaged with fruits and vegetables. Even if you live in a small apartment, you can still grow sprouts in a jar and lettuces, herbs, and vegetables in pots. There are always options. Kids love to grow food. They love the whole process, and watching plants grow and change is interesting and engaging. Just remember the effects may show up much later, so don't make any comments if the child doesn't eat the tomatoes that he has grown.

What Happens When the Kids are Out of the House?

All of this works great when you're home with your kids, where you have control over what's being served and when, but many parents ask the question: "What should we do when we're out of the house?" You're not going to be able to stop them (nor should you) from going to birthday parties where there are cupcakes, potato chips, and soda pop. You should not ridicule or put them down for being "weak" if they indulge. What's important is that the majority of the time you're surrounding them with healthy choices. Your kids will not fail, lapse, or "go off the wagon," or be condemned to a lifetime of struggling with obesity because of the occasional ice cream, pizza, or birthday cake. Junk food will inevitably trickle in, so don't make a big deal about it. For example, have birthday cake, go trick-or-treat-

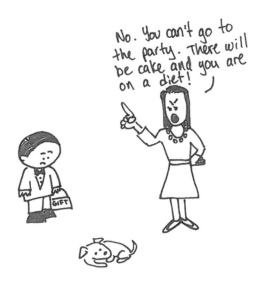

ing, and try grandma's cookies. When they go to a pizza party, don't single them out as not being allowed to eat any pizza or as being on a diet. To successfully enable this process, you need to get the junk food out of your own home, so a monthly survey, especially after holidays or special occasions, may be a good new habit.

School Lunches

Unfortunately, with very few exceptions, school cafeterias are not serving food of optimal nutrition or offering healthy choices on a regular basis. Kids are left to choose from processed, highly refined, empty-calorie foods, like microwaved pizza and deep-fried chicken nuggets with fries. But even though schools in general are not the healthiest places to eat, it's still okay for children to eat cafeteria food once a week or so. But when possible, packing a lunch and snack is always a better option, so we recommend that you usually pack your kids' lunches.

Here are some general guidelines, a checklist for packed lunches:

- No added sugar in any foods
- At least one fruit
- At least one vegetable
- At least one serving of protein, like unprocessed meat, chicken, fish, nuts, or eggs
- Water to drink
- A note saying "Have a nice day," or "I love you."

Do not be too worried about putting too much food in the lunch box. If it is all healthy and they are hungry, they will eat. If they aren't, they won't. They can use anything they didn't eat for snacks during after-school activities.

Do not judge the lunch you packed on how much is eaten or make comments about it to your kids. One great way to get your children involved in what they eat is to let them help shop for and prepare their lunches. Dr. Patricia loves to go to Whole Foods with her daughter. She'll say, "Choose one fruit and vegetable you want in your lunch," or "Let's choose some proteins." Make sure at least one fruit and one vegetable are in their lunch daily. Variety is key.

Here are some specific, simple, real-food solutions:

- Adding a raw fruit and a vegetable, like cut melon and carrots
- Chicken or shrimp salad
- Cut vegetables with hummus or guacamole
- Cut fresh fruit—rotate through seasons
- Mixed berry puree
- Hard-boiled eggs
- Pinwheels made of either turkey and cheese or roast beef and cheese
- Unsweetened applesauce
- Nut and seed trail mix
- Almond bread, Ezekiel bread (gluten free), or 100 percent whole-grain sandwiches made with peanut or almond butter and sliced strawberries, or roast beef, turkey, or chicken with hummus or guacamole, cheese, and pickles.
- String cheese

We recommend packing lunch and both a midmorning and an afternoon snack.

Also, we strongly recommend having a healthy snack waiting for your kids as soon as they get home from school. That's typically when your children's blood sugar levels will be low. Low blood sugar causes junk food cravings, so if you can have a healthy snack ready to go as soon as you pick them up or they walk through the door, it will stabilize their blood sugar and prevent severe junk food cravings.

Ideal snacks start with a fresh fruit and vegetable and could include:

- Celery or an apple with peanut butter
- Smoothies with fruit, chia seeds, protein powder, unsweetened almond milk, plain yogurt, and/or coconut water.
- Nut and seed trail mix
- Sliced fruit with plain yogurt—you can sweeten the yogurt with unsweetened applesauce and nuts.
- Cut vegetables, like carrots, celery, or other crispy veggies, with healthy dips like hummus or guacamole.
- Vegetable soups
- Sliced apples with cinnamon
- Omelet or frittata
- Meat and cheese pinwheels
- Ezekiel bread (gluten free) or 100 percent whole-grain with nut butter and a side of fruit
- Cauliflower nori sushi and miso soup
- Mini meatballs and fresh melon served with toothpicks
- Tomatoes and basil with mozzarella cheese on skewers—you can add balsamic vinaigrette

Please visit TheGabrielMethod.com/FitKids and DrRibasHealthClub .org/FitKids for recipes and other ideas.

Of course, packed lunches and snacks don't have to be confined to school. Making healthy to-go food is a good skill for you to develop and teach your children. You can prepare packed lunches for any outing. The same general health guidelines apply when your kids are at a friend's house or out with their friends:

- Pack water to drink.
- Make sure there's a fruit and vegetable on their plate for all meals and snacks when possible.
- Choose active play when making plans with friends—hikes, biking, sports, or games.

Most importantly, don't focus on trying to force kids to comply when they are out of the house. As they get used to what you are serving, have confidence that they will gravitate toward healthier foods. Also, have confidence and faith in your children to make healthy choices more often when not with you.

And if it's a special occasion, let them eat whatever they want and don't stress about it. Feel confident that everything else you're doing is making a major difference toward putting your kids back on track and getting them fitter, healthier, and most importantly, establishing healthy patterns for the rest of their lives.

Even though attitudes about food have to change, we don't want those attitudes to change at the expense of your social, cultural, or religious life. People have always associated food with celebration, but we guarantee you that our ancestors weren't celebrating sports carnivals or religious festivals with hot dogs, soda pop, or candy bars laden with corn syrup, hydrogenated vegetable oil, and food coloring. Celebrating achievements or holidays with food will always be wonderful, so celebrate with delicious, real foods when possible, whether you're at a restaurant or at home.

Your child's taste will change when you stop buying and serving sweetened and processed foods. By serving natural food, you will reset their taste-o-meter, and over time, they will gravitate toward more healthful foods.

In the end, it's never a good idea to give love, praise, or scorn based on if, or how much, the child eats. That is not your responsibility. Children need to feel loved and connected to you no matter what. Let them feel secure in your love, regardless of the food that they choose to eat.

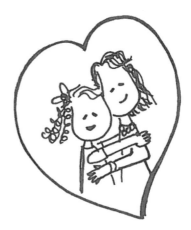

5

Soothing the Stress

What are some of the barriers to being healthier that your family is faced with? Is it having enough money to buy healthy food? Saying no to your children when they want fast food, and you are so tired from your day that the last thing you want to do is cook? Is it finding time to exercise? Is there a sick loved one at home or in the hospital? Are you battling your kids at bedtime?

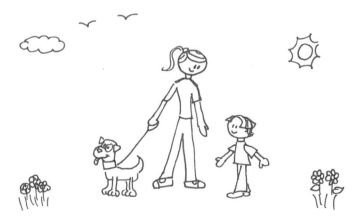

Whatever they are (and we're sure there are many), we all have many barriers to good health. One common barrier is stress. Reports have found that stress levels have increased up to 30 percent in the past thirty years, with young and low-income individuals affected the most.[1] Stress can overpower individuals, as well as a whole household. It can cause real medical problems, including obesity and emotional eating. Overeating is a coping mechanism many individuals use to deal with stress.[2] The relationship of stress and depression is well-known, and it can cause an increased emotional response to food, which makes normal eating patterns difficult and is often associated with weight gain.[3,4,5]

In order to better understand stress, let's start by discussing the Hierarchy of Needs, as developed by psychologist Abraham Maslow in the 1940s. Maslow's insights into which needs are most important help us to understand that your family's most basic physiological needs (water, food, shelter, sleep) must be met first, before anyone can stress or worry about things like friendship or self-esteem.

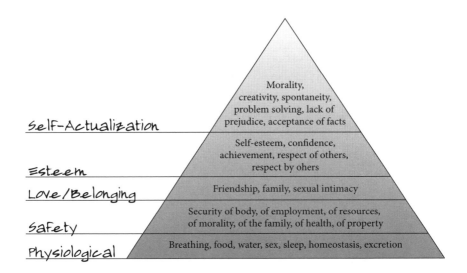

The stresses to consider first are the ones that make your children feel unsafe: bad health, abuse (emotional, physical, or sexual), and a lack of basic resources needed to keep them alive. For example, if you are sick and vomiting, the likelihood that you are worrying about improving your forehand in tennis is pretty slim. If a child is constantly in fear of being beaten up at school, he's probably not worrying about his grades and completing his homework on time. You can't concentrate on a conversation if you have to pee really badly. If you can't breathe, your body will deal with this urgent need first, before you can argue a point or paint a picture. There are many different types of stresses, all of which affect your children and the entire family.

The first way to deal with stress is to figure out where it is coming from. It is important to understand Maslow's Hierarchy of Needs and determine where your stressors fall on the pyramid. According to the American Psychological Association (APA), the top causes of stress for adults include:

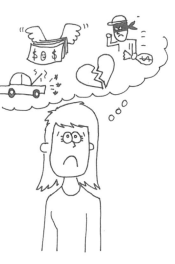

- Money
- Work
- The economy
- Family responsibilities
- Relationships
- Personal health concerns
- Housing costs
- Job stability
- Health problems affecting the family
- Personal safety

Once you identify the stressors in your life, understand that your child is experiencing these stressors too. According to the APA's Stress in America Findings, 91 percent of children in 2010 reported that they knew when a parent was stressed, despite nearly 70 percent of parents claiming that their stress had no impact on their children.[6]

According to the American Academy of Pediatrics and www.familyeducation.com, the top sources of stress for kids include:

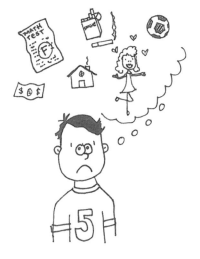

- Watching parents argue
- Pressure from school (grades, test taking, learning disabilities, and so on)
- Fighting with a friend or a sibling
- Not having enough privacy
- Not being good enough at sports
- Birth of a brother or sister (sibling rivalry)
- Moving to a new school
- Worrying about how their body is changing
- Marriage or remarriage of a parent
- Not having enough money[7]

Food Restriction and Dieting

Families often come to Dr. Patricia's practice as a last resort, already having tried many diets and feeling extremely stressed about their child's weight. Oftentimes, these obese children feel horribly guilty about their weight and, to add insult to injury, have been self-soothing by emotional eating. They are worried about what they eat and don't eat, and they feel badly about themselves if they don't exercise. They often feel powerless and vulnerable. When Dr. Patricia's team sees families or individuals actively overeating or engaged in emotional eating, there is generally an underlying problem bigger than just the types of foods they are eating. The enormous stress of being put on a diet makes many children feel like they might not get enough food, so they binge, hoard, and hide food from those restricting them and subsequently feel more guilt and shame. Parents think they are not trying hard enough, so they restrict more. This is a vicious cycle. If nothing else, please never put your child on a diet and never try to control portions. As you learned in chapters 3 and 4, offer a variety of nutritious choices and let children self-regulate their eating.

Another common source of stress for children can be bullying, particularly if a child is overweight. Bullying can cause a range of health issues—anxiety, depression, physical illness, mental anguish, sleeping problems, and headaches.[8] The Centers for Disease Control and Prevention (CDC) found that 23 percent of public schools reported bullying occurring on a regular basis, with more incidents reported for middle school students than for high school students.[9] Children can be cruel, especially to each other, and obese children take a lot of abuse from their peers and adults. Parents of overweight and obese children have rated bullying as their number one concern.[10] They are frequently the butt of jokes and receive snide, belittling comments and putdowns. Bullying alienates and marginalizes obese children, turning them into social outcasts, making matters worse for them and burdening them with feelings of shame and inadequacy.

Victims of bullying are more than six times more likely to be diagnosed with a serious illness or disorder than people who are not victims of bullying.[11] It can also make a child hypersensitive, seeing attacks and put-downs in even the most innocent of events. This is a serious issue and causes stress for many children, and it should not be taken lightly. In Dr. Patricia's practice, she recommends parents and children read the book *Wonder* by R J Palacio to help put things in perspective.

In order to deal with bullies, the American Academy of Pediatrics[12] recommends that you teach your child to do the following:

- Not react to the bully.
- Look the bully in the eye.
- If the bully continues, be assertive—stand tall and stay calm.
- Walk away.

Teach your child how to say in a firm voice:

- "I don't like what you are doing."
- "Please do *not* talk to me like that."
- "Why would you say that?"

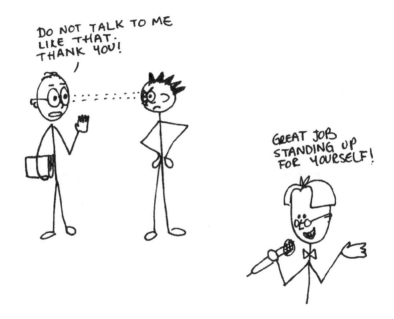

Parents should follow up with their school to let teachers and administrators know of the problem and should be knowledgeable of the school's procedures on how to deal with the situation. Seek counseling for the child if it becomes a recurring problem and above all, make sure your child feels safe at school.

Ideally, we want to be aware of the stressors in our lives and do what we can to minimize them and decrease their harm. It is impossible to have zero stress in our lives, but we can teach by example, developing healthy habits as ways to overcome it.

Here are some ideas adapted from the American Academy of Pediatrics[13] and us for reducing stress:

- Figure out what the problem is and work to make it manageable (people who try to fix their problems tend to be emotionally healthier than those who don't).
- Break up big work into small pieces so it is less overwhelming.
- Make lists of what you need to do.
- Avoid things that bring you down.
- Let some things go.
- Practice mind-body relaxation techniques, like meditation, visualization, yoga, tai chi, or qigong.
- Journal.
- Exercise.
- Share your feelings with the family. Caution: parents should not burden their children with their problems.
- Take a warm bath.
- Get a massage.
- Sleep well.

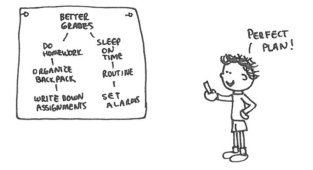

Once you've adopted the principles related to mealtimes in chapter 4, you can help overcome stress by having family-centered meals where children feel safe and comfortable sharing their day's highs and lows without worrying about what or how much they are eating. This can offer you a lot of insight into your child's day and help release their daily tensions. Sometimes discussions with loved ones can help dissipate a problem and allow children to learn how to verbalize their feelings and emotions and find solutions. Oftentimes, parents can share life experiences and cultural or religious stories that empower their children to solve their own problems and give them a framework or new perspective on their problems, helping them feel less alone or overwhelmed.

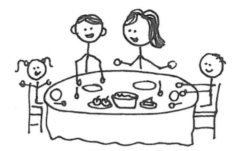

Making mealtimes pleasant can provide a great anchor for your child's well-being. Family members assembling and supporting one another can make children feel very protected.

One study found that the most powerful tool associated with lower body mass index (BMI), for both adults and children, was family meals eaten together at the dinner table.[14] One reason for this may be that family members can share their thoughts on the day and enjoy a meal together without stressors and distractions (like the television) affecting their interaction or their body's cues for being satisfied.

Regular exercise is also a great way to help children and parents get rid of stress. It should be fun. Place a football in Grandma's hands, or put Dad in a tutu or wig for family dancing. Laugh, tickle, play tag, go to the park, or play together with glow-in-the-dark Frisbees. While you move and bond, see the daily stresses melt off your children's shoulders—and yours.

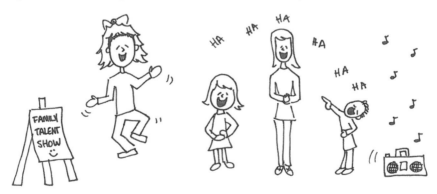

Finally, adequate sleep is a huge factor in managing stress and one that is often overlooked, as we will discuss in chapter 7. Creating and adhering to regular bedtime routines is imperative for children and adults. Reading books and practicing visualizations together can be great for bonding and de-stressing.

These activities help enrich intimacy, bonding experiences, and friendship in the home and can satisfy your child's need for a deeper connection.

Children, like adults, have enough stress in their lives. As we've seen, some are more avoidable than others, and it serves us to understand stress from many different angles. One stress that can be harder to avoid than others is the toxic stress that comes from pollution and chemicals in the environment. Even so, there is a lot that we can do to help ourselves and our children minimize its effects. The next chapter explains some of the things you can do.

6

Protecting Your Child
from a Toxic World

In addition to the mental stressors that our children face, we also need to look at environmental stressors with respect to obesity.

Environmental toxins can stress our bodies in significant ways that are difficult for the eye to see. You don't have to live next to a chemical plant to be exposed to high levels of toxicity. Even if there were no other environmental stresses, like those from emotional violence, abuse, general negativity, or nutritional deprivation, the chemical stress that we're exposed to alone could have an enormous effect on obesity.[1]

When toxic chemicals are introduced into our bodies, we have to deal with them somehow. We have to detoxify these chemicals by changing their structure or breaking them down. The main organ for doing this is the liver. Now, if you've ever seen a liver, it looks like a big, brown lump, but it's actually the largest organ in the body after your skin; it's the body's largest gland, and some say it rivals the brain in complexity. But as miraculous as the liver is, it can only do so much at any one time. Detoxification is only one of its many functions, and when it's overwhelmed, the body still has to do something with all those toxins. So what does it do?

It stores toxic chemicals in fat cells. Why? Because fat is a great chemical cushion. It's like bubble wrap, isolating and containing toxic chemicals until the liver is ready to deal with them. And the more toxicity in your body, the more fat you need. In fact, one study showed that some people are storing at least eight hundred different toxic chemicals in an average fat cell at any one time.[2]

In addition, a 2012 study published in *Time Magazine* reported that exposure to air pollution during pregnancy was found to be associated with heavier birth weights.[3] Children born to these highly exposed mothers had a nearly 80 percent greater risk of becoming obese when compared with those born to mothers who were not as highly exposed to air toxins.

But it's not just air pollution we have to consider. Toxins are everywhere, in things as seemingly innocent as the plastic containers in our kitchen. These days, you can find the plastic additive BPA everywhere because this colorless solid is used in the manufacturing of polycarbonate polymers, including many of those clear plastics used to make drink bottles. Unfortunately, BPA mimics the properties of various hormones and affects many of our bodies' regulatory systems.

In 2010, the US Food and Drug Administration warned of possible BPA-associated hazards "on the brain, behavior, and prostate gland in fetuses, infants, and young children."[4] But more pertinent to our immediate concerns are the results of a study published in the *Journal of the American Medical Association*. Lead researcher, Leonardo Trasande of the New York University of Medicine, and his colleagues:

Reviewed data on body mass index (BMI) and BPA exposure (determined by measuring the chemical in urine) in 2,838 children aged 6 through 19, who participated in the government's National Health and Nutrition Examination Surveys (NHANES) between 2003 and 2008. About 34 percent of the children were overweight and 18 percent were obese.

Those in the highest quartile of BPA exposure also had the highest rate of obesity, at 22.3 percent, while those with the lowest levels of the chemical in their urine were least likely to be obese, at 10 percent. That's more than a doubling of obesity risk among those with the highest BPA exposure."[5]

This study shows that, along with diet and physical activity, parents need to consider environmental factors as another contributor to their children's health problems and a potential threat to their children's well-being.

We recommend minimizing contact with food wrapped or contained in BPA plastics, most of which, inevitably, will be processed food. And if you think that the wrapping is potentially harmful, consider the contents. As we've already noted, there's very little solid information on what a lot of these substances, particularly in the form of food additives (mentioned in chapter 3), might be doing to your or your children's bodies.

In addition to chemicals found in our air, food, containers, and cookware, we are also affected by our medications that as a culture, we've become increasingly dependent upon. According to Dr. Joel Fuhrman, all medications are toxic to the body in some way, increasing our overall toxic load and stress response. Some medications, like certain antidepressants and steroids, directly cause weight gain.[6]

In Dr. Patricia's practice, she critically evaluates every medication each patient is taking and works with the family and prescribing physicians to eliminate or wean them from as many as possible. Her team tries to reduce the use of many of the psychiatric and behavioral medicines children take regularly, particularly if they are not necessarily helping behavior. Parents should not arbitrarily stop any prescription medications but should work with the prescribing doctor to see if it is possible to safely eliminate or decrease them.

Given that many people just don't have the option of moving to a pristine or chemical-free environment, drinking lots of filtered water is probably the easiest and most practical way to clean out accumulated environmental poisons. David Wolfe, raw food guru, likes to refer to water as the "solution to pollution." In fact, there is a common expression Dr. Patricia's vet uses, which is "Dilution is the solution to pollution." He uses this when flushing out wounds, but it also works on the inside of our bodies.

Eliminating chemical- and sugar-laden liquids and drinking pure water are two of the most important factors in weight loss. BPA-free bottled water or filtered water is the way to go. It's really important that the water be clean and free of chlorine, because the chlorine that kills unfriendly bacteria in the water supply and in pipes is the same chlorine that will kill the friendly, essential bacteria in your gut, which you need to get the maximum nutrition from your food. If you filter your own water, check your water supply to see if carbon filtration is adequate to purify it. Chlorine is there for a reason. If you take it out without getting rid of what it was killing, you may get sick. Ideally, reverse osmosis is necessary to purify your water effectively.

We recommend you offer water to your children first thing in the morning and throughout the day. Just make sure that your child (and you, for that matter) stay hydrated all day. Remember that water is also a great way to flush out the toxins that leach out of your fat while you're losing weight. An easy way for children to know if they are getting enough water is simply to look in the toilet bowl after urinating. If the urine looks dark yellow, they probably need to drink more water. A common exception to this is if they're on vitamin B supplementation, as B vitamins tend to give urine a bright yellow color. An adequately hydrated child's urine should be almost clear. That's the sign that he or she is getting enough water.

Water is, of course, not the only way to fight toxins in your environment. Here are our recommendations for dealing with the environmental stressors in our lives:

- Get out in nature whenever possible and breathe fresh air.
- Eat organic produce and grass-fed organic meats.
- Grow your own food (if you can).
- Buy locally grown, spray-free food from a farmer's market.
- Eat superfoods, like spirulina and chlorella (which help to counter heavy metal poisoning).[7]
- Eat lots of greens and other foods, like fruits and vegetables, rich in antioxidants.
- Drink lots of fresh green juices, especially wheatgrass juice.
- Take probiotics, as they will help support a healthy immune system.
- Use household cleaning products that are made of natural ingredients.
- Avoid exposure to secondhand smoke.

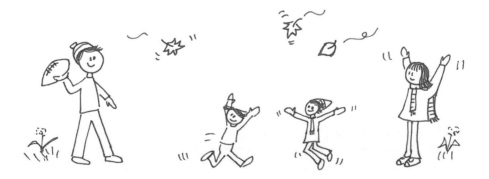

Aside from chemical stressors that seem to be an inevitable part of modern civilization, there's another significant stress that has arisen as a result of modern lifestyle choices. That stress is sleep deprivation, and it's one of the least acknowledged stresses that contribute to obesity, as you'll learn in the next chapter.

7

Nourish Your Child with Sleep

Are you trying to squeeze too much into each day? Do you have a hard time getting your kids to go to sleep? Do one or more family members snore? Is sleep a priority? A good night's sleep is vital to being healthy. We all fill our days and nights with too much (even both of us admit to trying to fit too much into each day).

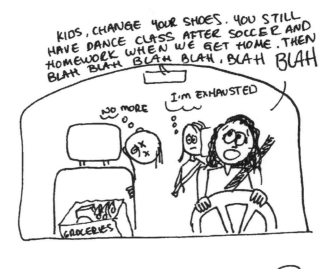

All of this leads to a poor quality of sleep, and even to sleep deprivation, which is stressful on the body. Our body clocks have become more and more detached from natural rhythms and natural cycles. This lack of connection, between what our bodies need and what we force them to do, contributes to the stresses that we put ourselves and our children through.

According to the CDC, more than one quarter of the United States population suffers from insufficient sleep.[1] While adults generally need eight hours of sleep a night, more than 20 percent of the population reported that they regularly get less than six hours a night.[2] Sleep deprivation is associated with decreased alertness, memory impairment, increased stress, and poor quality of life, as well as chronic diseases, including diabetes and depression.[3] In addition, sleep deprivation can be a big barrier to weight loss. Getting enough sleep is often recognized as an essential part of a healthy lifestyle and for promoting disease prevention.

Natural sleep cycles vary. If we followed the rhythms of the natural world, we'd be more active in the summer when we have more available daylight, and in the winter, we'd be less active and sleep more. But modern society forces us to be at work or school regardless of what our bodies need, and artificial lighting extends our waking hours and activities beyond what our ancestors adapted to for tens of thousands of years. The effects of this are bad enough for adults, but even more significant for children. Even minor changes in sleep duration can negatively affect children's ability to learn and concentrate.[4]

Getting children to go to bed at regular hours and get enough sleep isn't just an important way to preserve parental sanity. Sufficient and regular sleep is vital to your child's health, and yes, there is a link between sleep and childhood obesity. One study found that children who are not getting the recommended amount of sleep per night suffer from obesity *four times* more often than children

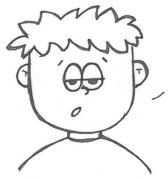

I'M SLEEPY...
UMM...
OR MAYBE
HUNGRY?...

who get adequate sleep.[5] The authors concluded that sleep has an important impact on metabolism, and too little sleep will slow down metabolism and result in excess weight. To elaborate, sleep deprivation disrupts levels of ghrelin and leptin, two hormones that regulate hunger and appetite. "When the body craves sleep, it interprets it as hunger, causing leptin levels to crash and ghrelin levels to spike; this in turn, seems to trigger overeating and may also signal the body to cling to fat stores more tenaciously."[6] This was found to be especially true among young children who are still growing and need more sleep for proper growth and development.

Any lack of sleep, interrupted sleep, or poor quality of sleep creates stress on a child's body.[7]

Obese children, just like obese adults, are more likely to suffer from interrupted sleep, which can affect your child's mental functioning and which will, in turn, increase obesity.[8] This means that obese people are more likely to have sleep apnea, which can impair their mental functioning cognitively and negatively affect development.[9]

So, how much sleep do your children need? Here is a guide produced by the American Academy of Pediatrics (AAP) and the CDC to help you evaluate if your child is sleeping enough:

Between birth and 2 months, children need 12–18 hours of sleep
Between 3 and 11 months, children need 14–15 hours of sleep
Between 1–3 years, children need 12–14 hours of sleep
Between 3–5 years, children need 11–13 hours of sleep
Between 5–10 years, children need 10–11 hours of sleep
Between 10–17 years, children and teenagers need 8.5–9.5 hours
    of sleep [10]

To promote regular sleep, you can practice good sleep hygiene techniques, which are different practices necessary to quality nighttime sleep. The most prominent example of these is maintaining a regular sleep and wake pattern. These bedtime routine guidelines, adapted from the AAP, can help.[11]

Bedtime Routines

- **Develop bedtime rituals.** These are powerful cues that it is time for bed. Some examples include: reading a story, putting away stuffed animals, brushing teeth, or saying good night to the animals. These signal that it is time to change, brush teeth, and get ready for bed.
- **Set limits on attention-getting behaviors at night.** Recurring nighttime waking can become a social habit when these patterns are reinforced. Be sure not to encourage these types of behaviors often.

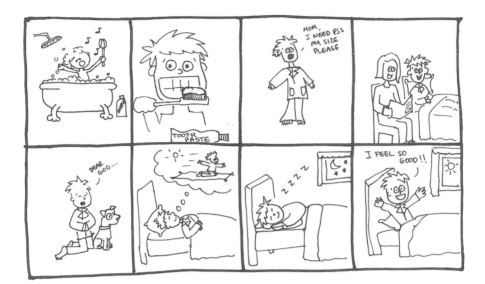

- **Pay attention to the sleep environment.** A cool, dark, quiet room is ideal. Pay attention to anything that can affect sleep, such as lighting, noise, favorite toys, and bedding.
- **Limit time in bed.** Children should only sleep in their bed, and once awake, should be up and out of bed. They should not watch television, play video games, or do homework in bed.
- **Establish consistent waking times.** These should be consistent seven days a week, which will help establish good sleep rhythms and help children adhere to bedtimes.
- **Avoid caffeinated drinks.** Caffeine should be avoided from the afternoon into evening, as it is a stimulant and will make going to bed even more difficult. We don't recommend any caffeine for children
- **Avoid medications to help your child sleep.** These can affect alertness during the day, making sleeping difficult. Also, some medications can cause nightmares.
- **Discourage excessive evening fluids.** This can cause bed-wetting and reawakening. Let your children drink to their thirst, but no more.
- **Chart your child's progress.** Use praise for successful, quiet nights. You can make a star chart to track their progress and reward them once they fill it up to encourage successful nights.

- **Consider medical problems.** Sleep apnea, pain, allergies, or asthma can all disrupt sleep and make consistent sleep difficult. Snoring can be a sign of sleep apnea and should be medically evaluated.
- **Make the bedroom a sleep-only zone.** This means, at the very least, the bed should only be used for sleeping, not studying or playing. A few stuffed animals are fine in bed, but remove other toys, games, televisions, computers, mobile devices, and radios if your child is having trouble falling asleep.

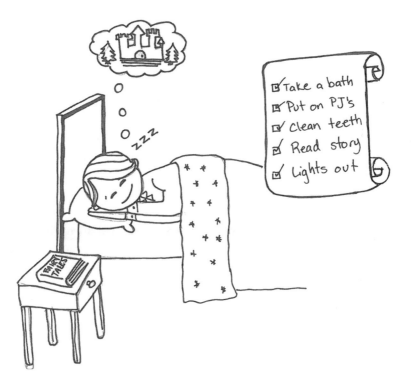

Sleep Apnea and Weight Gain

Nightly snoring in children can be a symptom of a potentially life-threatening sleep disorder called *sleep apnea*. If your child snores every once in a while, that is normal, but if they snore often or nightly, they should see a doctor. (Note: not all children with sleep apnea snore.) This condition happens when breathing is interrupted during sleep. This interruption might be caused by congestion due to allergies, illness, mouth breathing, or adenoids. While experiencing sleep apnea, your child can literally start to asphyxiate. His or her body then partially wakes up to restore breathing, thus, interrupting rapid eye movement (REM) sleep, which is vital for good health. Instead of nights of normal, uninterrupted sleep, apnea sufferers' sleep cycles become a series of microsleeps, leaving the sufferer not only sleep deprived, but also oxygen deprived and exhausted.[12] Side effects of interrupted sleep include: increased blood pressure, increased heart size, heart attack, heart disease, and stroke. Patients wake up unrefreshed. Adults can have life-threatening accidents because they fall asleep at the wheel or on the job. Children can fall asleep at school and have difficulty concentrating, which ultimately interferes with school performance.

Fortunately, the solutions for sleep apnea or apnea-like symptoms are relatively simple. Allergy testing to reduce mucous, examination of air passages, breathing coaches, altering bedding, and changing sleeping positions can all help. Perhaps a chicken or the egg thing, weight loss, in and of itself, can also alleviate *obstructive sleep apnea* (OSA). In more severe cases of sleep apnea, your doctor can prescribe surgery or a continuous positive airway pressure (CPAP) machine, which is a mask connected to an air pump that keeps air flowing directly into the nose all night long. A variety of mask models are available to make them as comfortable for your child as possible.

Regardless of what might or might not be contributing to weight gain in children, if children snore, they should be evaluated by a doctor to see if they have OSA, which can also cause high blood pressure, seizures, poor school performance, and, in extreme cases, sudden death.[13] So please don't assume that snoring is harmless. We strongly recommend that children be evaluated for OSA through a sleep study.

Dr. Patricia has had many patients with OSA. A few resolved their symptoms after losing weight, while others had to have it treated *before* they could lose weight. One child, Jenny, had her tonsils removed when she was three years old, and no one ever asked if the snoring she had previously suffered from had returned. By the time I saw her in her teens, she was sleeping sitting up in a chair at night to breathe. She had high blood pressure, was on medications for poor behavior, was suffering from seizures, and was failing classes at school. I immediately ordered a sleep study, and my suspicions were verified.

Sleep studies normally involve monitoring a patient with support equipment to evaluate their oxygen levels during unaided sleep. But in this case, Jenny's OSA was so bad that the study had to be stopped early because her oxygen levels became so critically low that she had to be given oxygen. She immediately started using a CPAP machine, and her blood pressure improved, her seizures stopped, and she began to wean gradually from her behavioral medications. Unfortunately, she'd grown up feeling tired all of the time and thinking she was mentally challenged and couldn't learn at school, so some psychological damage had already been done. You don't want this to happen to your child, so we recommend that if you have the slightest concern, consult with a physician to address this problem as soon as possible. The heavier a child is, the more likely they are to have sleep apnea, so if your child is 55 pounds or more overweight, we strongly suggest a sleep study.

Jon also had life-threatening sleep apnea, but it went away after he lost weight. Jon used a CPAP machine and felt it was an essential component to his weight loss. Today, when Jon works with clients, he frequently recommends sleep studies. This is a point we can't emphasize strongly enough.

The association between sleep duration and weight gain is clear, and the impact of insufficient sleep on obesity risk is even greater in children than in adults.[14] Significant associations have been documented between children who slept less at night and long-term obesity and higher adult BMI values.[15]

Your children's bodies are constantly growing and changing. Good sleep will establish patterns that will last their whole lives. One of the most important patterns that you can establish is active, physical engagement with the world, so that your children can respond to the many physical challenges that they'll face in life in the most pristine of environments.

One way for your children to get better sleep is by being more active. Regular exercise has been linked to better, sounder sleep, and as a bonus, an active body is far less likely to be overweight than an inactive one.[16,17]

8

How to Foster an Active Lifestyle

Exercise is an important part of a healthy lifestyle, and achieving its benefits can be easier and more fun than you might think. Regular exercise is one of the best ways to help reduce and cope with stress. Regular physical activity in childhood helps improve strength, builds healthy muscles, reduces anxiety and stress, and helps improve self-esteem.[1] Other benefits include reducing the risk of chronic diseases like diabetes and certain types of cancers, improving students' academic performance, and improving mood. Exercise helps individuals be healthier, have better behavior, and have a more positive sense of well-being.

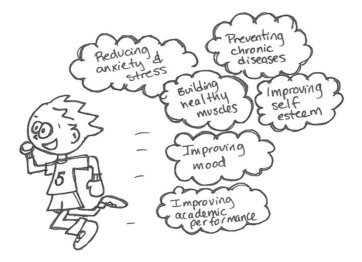

This sense of well-being is especially critical for obese children, who typically have lower self-esteem than their normal-weight counterparts. Many studies have found that regular physical activity helps improve children's confidence, self-esteem, and level of achievement, and also reduces depression symptoms.[2,3] Many researchers have found that the positive effects of exercise tend to make children feel better about themselves, which helps them do better in school, pay more attention, and sleep better. This is a powerful tool for improving your child's health, reducing his or her stress, and improving his or her mood.[4]

It is universally recommended that children ages five to seventeen get sixty minutes of physical activity a day.[5,6,7] Ideally, this should be in the form of simply playing, just kids being kids. Unfortunately, many children are not getting anywhere close to these recommendations. A 2013 Institute of Medicine report found that half of the children in the United States are not meeting the physical activity guidelines of sixty minutes a day.[8] A big concern, this report noted, is that less than 10 percent of elementary, middle, and high schools provide daily physical education.

While we know we should all be moving more, the fact is that the neighborhoods our children live in today are nothing like those of our parents. Data from fifty countries and more than fifty million children show that kids' fitness was improving up until 1970, before a rapid decline, which is still continuing, occurred. According to Professor Tim Olds, Director of the Kids Eat, Kids Play National Survey,[9] kids today are up to 15 percent less fit than their parents were at the same age, and kids are 20 percent heavier than their parents were.[10] We can't blame the kids for these statistics, though. What chance does a kid have of burning excess calories and building active muscle mass in a neighborhood where there are no parks to play in or where the perception of danger, or even urban sprawl, is such that you feel you must drive your kids everywhere, instead of letting them walk or catch public transport? And even if there are safe parks to play in, it seems that kids today are more interested in the virtual realities offered through television, computer games, and the Internet than they are in nature, playing in real grass or among real trees and nature.

An interesting fact that has emerged from the study Growing Up in Australia is that more children are spending more time inside doing sedentary activities related to obesity, like watching television.[11] Nearly 50 percent of four- to five-year-olds watch more than two hours of television per day, which is more than the time spent walking, running, or doing any other exercise or activity. Television alone increases the likelihood for obesity, impaired social behavior, poor school performance, and higher rates of violence.[12] In fact, children who have a television in their bedroom are twice as likely to be obese compared with those without a television in their room.[13] So if your child has a television in the bedroom, you might want to consider relocating it.

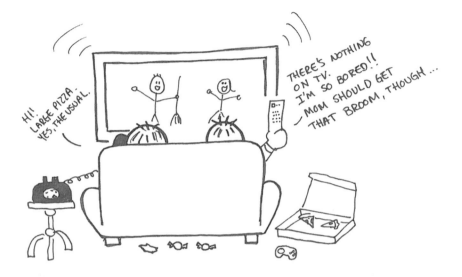

"We've just reached rock bottom in terms of levels of inactivity," said Professor Tim Olds. "We simply couldn't be more inactive than we are at the moment. We have so many self-opening doors, so many remote controls, so many labor-saving devices, so many cars driving kids to school. I think it is true to say that convenience is killing us. Convenience is making us fat. If you live in a household where physical activity is the norm, where Dad goes cycling, and Mum plays tennis or goes jogging and the whole family goes swimming, and so forth, it's something that becomes a bit like eating with a knife and fork. It just becomes second nature to the child; it's part of the thing to do.[14]

We know that children who are physically active are much less likely to be overweight. Exercise is a great way to promote cardiovascular fitness; increase coordination, flexibility, and muscle strength; and generally improve health and mental well-being. There are many well-known, well-publicized, and highly promoted benefits to exercise that go beyond any question of weight loss. The problem is most people think they cannot exercise frequently because they do not have enough time, money, and space. Fortunately, you don't need to have that much time, money, and space because there is a solution that can work for almost any family.

First, we need to understand that children are motivated differently than adults. Adults will put themselves through repetitive exercises for many reasons, like wanting to get into shape so they can get more dates or fit into a wedding dress or because they want to run a marathon or enter a competition. Adults are willing to undergo short-term pain for long-term gain. And many adults actually like repetitive exercise. Kids, however, often do not enjoy these types of activities and prefer more fun activities like playing, chasing, and competition. Exercise should be fun! Let children follow their own ideas and do what they enjoy.

Most children want to have fun and they want to be involved in an activity—whether mental or physical—that is entertaining. Most kids like skill-based activities, and since the first thing that comes into people's minds when you say "skill-based physical activities" is sports, we'll talk about it first.

The general rule with sports is that you should treat them like food choices: offer a range of healthy options within your means. No matter whether you live in a city or in the country, or whether it's the height of summer or the depths of winter, there are likely to be a number of different sports or activities offered in

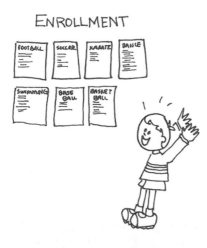

your local area. In fact, part of the charm of having different seasons is that they can inspire us to try different things at different times of the year, adding variety to our physical activities and experiences. Give your kids a taste of various activities, and let them guide you. If they like it, if it's fun for them, they'll do it. There are all sorts of reasons that children like some sports more than others.

Give them the space to try various things before they settle on something that they like. In the end, let your kids know that you're behind their choices,

including the choice not to do sports. Give them the space to try a new activity and be open-minded. Let them stop if it doesn't suit them. Sports, like food, should never be forced. Forcing children to participate in sports just creates unnecessary stress. Because there is something to be said for having them follow through on a commitment, you might have them finish the session and then simply not sign up for additional ones. If they at least finish a certain number of sessions, you'll know that they've really given it a chance.

Dealing with the mental, emotional, and nutritional factors of weight gain should go a long way toward increasing a child's desire for physical movement. The good news is that even children who are not athletically inclined can find physical activities that they love to do and will do, without any outside encouragement needed. And this brings us back to the concept of incidental exercise. Any type of extra movement is encouraged. Try parking farther away from the store, gardening outside, walking or biking instead of driving a car, and taking the stairs instead of the elevator, whenever you can. All of these add up and help your family become more active and healthy.

Kids who are less inclined to participate in organized sports can find other ways to be extremely active. Riding bikes, skateboarding, jumping rope, playing games outdoors, hiking, fishing, and gardening are all wonderful, natural ways for kids to balance their mental and physical health and to play and enjoy themselves. Walking to school will also contribute to good health as long as children aren't stopping at a convenience store to fill up on junk food on the way home!

Children with special needs can be a particular challenge when it comes to exercise, but try thinking outside the box and use unconventional, fun methods to get them to be more active. Some of Dr. Patricia's most challenging cases are children with autism, who can be particularly difficult to motivate to move more.

In one case, Benjamin, a teen with special needs, wouldn't leave the house, so Dr. Patricia and her team started by just getting him to play his video games and toys outside. In another case, the family tried gardening with a child, Suzanne, and she was able to figure out how to pull weeds and put them into the trash can. The father was so excited with this accomplishment that he suggested they move the trash can closer to the girl. The mom said, no, they should put it farther away. She was actually exercising! Finally, a third patient, Thomas, loved karate movies. So, while he watched the *Karate Kid* movie, he would copy the moves and be active. Using an unconventional approach, we had Thomas's mom show him an hour of the movies three times a week, and he actually got a great work out while Dr. Patricia and her team continued to find other ways to get him to play outside.

Children with spina bifida or other orthopedic conditions might benefit from working with a physical therapist who knows what the child can and cannot do and what areas he or she needs to strengthen. In essence, don't be discouraged if your child can't do conventional exercises. Brainstorm, and we're sure you can come up with different, fun ways to get him or her moving more.

Besides fresh air and extra space to run around, the outdoors provides something that's usually unavailable indoors—sunshine. Sunshine can play an important role in weight loss. For starters, increasing levels of sunshine signal that spring is coming, and with it, the promise of an end to the famine of winter and the coming abundance. Sunshine also increases levels of a group of hormones called *melancortins*, which increase the brain's sensitivity to the hormone leptin, the master hormone we keep talking about that determines the amount of fat on your body.[15] Sunshine is also the best way to get vitamin D, which is essential for a lot of body processes, including bone and teeth formation. From a weight-loss perspective, vitamin D reduces inflammation and the hormones that cause inflammation, which in turn affect the chemistry of obesity.[16,17,18]

The great thing about sunshine is that it's free. Your child only needs about ten to fifteen minutes of exposure to sunshine every day to get the full benefit. We understand that seasons change and that where you live, being outdoors might not always be an option. Fortunately, your kids don't have to be out-doors to be active.

When the weather is not cooperating (especially during the winter months when it is too dark or cold outside), then problem solve and get creative. You'll be amazed by all the activities you can do indoors, when it is rainy or cold, that do not require equipment or large areas. Here are some ideas for getting your family moving:

Indoor Activities for Rainy or Cold Days

- Dance.
- Play hide-and-go-seek.
- Follow a workout video (If you can, do it with your teens, who may especially enjoy this.)
- Play Simon Says with exercises.
- Practice hula-hooping.
- Jump rope.

- Imitate animals: bear crawl, hop like a bunny, alligator walk, crab walk, jump high like a kangaroo, spin like the Tasmanian devil, run like the roadrunner, fly like a bird flapping its wings, or frog jump (great for younger children).
- Play duck, duck, goose.
- Dance the hokey-pokey.
- Wheelbarrow with a partner.
- Stretch: touch your toes, be a flamingo, have an elephant trunk, pull your elbow behind your head with your other arm, or circle your arms.
- Make an indoor obstacle course.
- Play musical chairs.
- Practice balance activities: stand on one foot, stand on one toe, or do handstands.
- Have a pillow fight.
- Play tag.

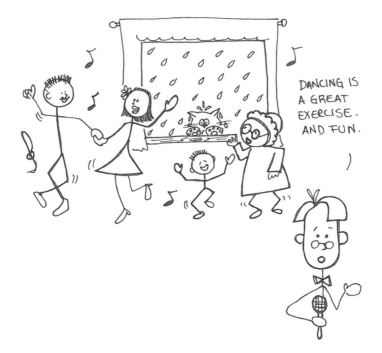

Don't get stuck on the idea that exercise can only come in the form of organized sports. In fact, we would advise that you avoid the word *exercise* altogether. Natural exercises are fun, and we included many in the indoor activity suggestions above. Never talk to your kids about "burning calories," "burning off that food," or "burning fat." Just talk about "playing," "racing," and "hiding." Try family activities together, such as rock climbing, hiking, and bike rides. Go on walks with your kids to find bunnies or frogs or to pick flowers. Carry a basket to collect shells from the beach or rocks you may find. Wear gloves and pick up trash or leaves together.

Many studies demonstrate that short, intense exercise sessions have a real, positive effect on health.[19,20] Some even claim that you only need small periods of intense exercise to gain most of the benefits of exercise.[21] For example, if you have an indoor bicycle and you peddle all out for five minutes, you'll stimulate your body to a point where the effect of that exercise will last for hours. The benefits of this high intensity interval training (HIIT) exercise include: increasing strength, endurance, oxygen intake capacity, and metabolism, as well as improving heart function. The most prominent type of this is Tabata regime training, a version of HIIT which was the first to use short periods of intense exercises (twenty seconds of exercise followed by ten seconds of rest, repeated continuously for four minutes) and was found to be the most effective form of exercise for weight loss.[22,23]

High intensity exercises are effective because our bodies are set up for survival. The fight-or-flight response is essentially what the HIIT exercises are mimicking, so those quick bursts of exercise represent an attack where your body has to respond quickly. For example, if a bear were to attack you, you wouldn't suddenly decide to do a forty-minute power walk; you would immediately run like the wind. And if you were swimming and saw a shark's fin, you wouldn't suddenly decide to do a lot of slow laps back to your boat, either. It

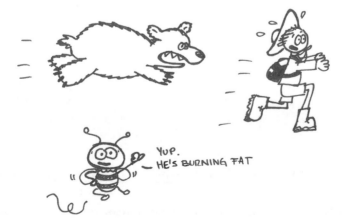

would be ten seconds, twenty seconds of all-out effort; it would be life and death, and then it would be over, one way or another.

That type of intense experience sets up dramatic changes in your body and will literally cause your body to burn fat. Instinctually, your body will do all it can to get out of danger *in a hurry*. Remember, it's about the hormonal environment that your body needs to create in order to survive.

You might not burn many calories in that thirty-second burst, but that's not the point. (Don't forget, we do not support the calories in and calories out notion, anyway.) The point is that thirty seconds of acute, immediate, all-out exertion is enough to set up a hormonal change that will put a body into fat-burning mode. If you put your child's body into that sort of acute stress situation a couple of times a week, it will burn fat, the effect will continue, and the child will lose weight.

This explains, in terms of weight loss, why short bursts of intense activity are as effective, if not even more so, as hours of other types of exercise. And here's the best part: you can do this right in your own home, with no equipment needed.

For many, HIIT can be a more realistic alternative than time-consuming, moderate-intensity training. Especially for inactive individuals, this can be the best start to get your body moving and used to regular exercise. An additional benefit is that it is much more practical and excuse free, since anyone can find ten minutes a day to move. Dr. Patricia's patients often excel at these types of workouts in her Fit Club program, an after-school and summer exercise program Dr. Patricia has been running since 2009. Run by her lead fitness trainer, Brandon Farmer, Fit Club incorporates these quick bursts of exercise into a circuit workout for children of different age groups and turns them into a game, coupled with cooking demonstrations, prizes, and healthy snacks. Some examples of games played to simulate the fight-or-flight response include relay races, dodge ball, tag, water-balloon fights, and sharks and minnows.

Not only does this mix up their workout, but it also makes it fun and exciting and produces great results. 2010 data from Fit Club (the official name of Dr. Patricia's organization) shows that 87 percent of participants decreased their BMI using these methods, and statistically significant improvements were found across the board in fitness scores (including sit-ups, push-ups, sit-and-reach, and the mile walk or run). While we recommend that children get sixty minutes of physical activity a day, we support the notion that intervals and quick bursts of exercise can have great benefits and should be incorporated to increase stamina and fat burning. Often HIIT exercises are a good place to start when trying to begin to incorporate exercise into your children's daily routine.

HIIT Workout Examples

As we said, simply playing an all-out intense game of tag, tickle tag, or sharks and minnows, or chasing your kids up and down the stairs of an apartment building for five minutes (remember, you only need to go all out for ten to twenty seconds at a time) is an effective start to burning fat and building muscle.[24] Not only is this great exercise, but it's also fun and it creates bonding. Kids just love being chased, especially by their parents. They're often faster than you are, so it gives them the impression, however brief, that they are empowered and have the upper hand, while at the same time feeling safe because it's all in good fun. Their body feels like it's being chased by a predator and will get the message that to stay safe it needs to get faster and stronger.

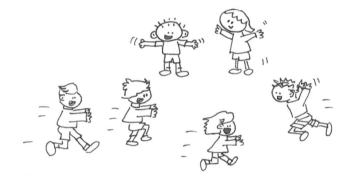

The great thing about this sort of play is that it incorporates the element of surprise. And it's exactly that surprise response that we want. You can't predict when the attack will happen. You can't predict how the game will go. This replicates the response to fight-or-flight threats in nature.

Here are some fun, healthy ways to do high-intensity interval training. These are intense, quick-burst activities that you can do with your kids:

- Pillow fights
- NERF gun battles
- Paintball battles
- Chases in the park
- Tag
- Tickle wars
- Races for rewards
- Frisbee

- Basketball
- Jumping on a trampoline
- Swimming pool and water games
- Sharks and minnows (in the pool or on land)

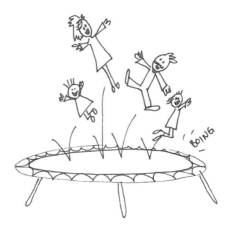

For those (possibly teenagers or parents) who want to try more intense Tabatas, here are some body weight exercises to try. Remember the correct Tabata form: each individual exercise is done for twenty seconds with a ten-second rest, repeating this a total of eight times over four minutes. For example, your kids can do jumping jacks for twenty seconds with a ten-second break, for a total of four minutes of jumping jacks. Ideally, the first round of jumping will be intense, and they want to try to do as many repetitions in the last round as they did in the first.

- Run in place
- Push-ups
- Squats
- Sit-ups
- Lunges
- Jumping jacks

Be sure kids have the correct form when doing the exercises listed above. Some notes and further description to help them out include:

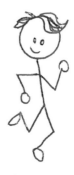

- **Run in place:** Stay in one spot while running as fast as you can. Make sure to bring your knees up close to your chest, and do not forget to pump your arms. If your left knee is coming up toward your chest, your right arm will be up, and vise versa. Also, keep your chin up and back flat, as you do not want to be bending over.
- **Push-ups:** Place both your hands flat on the ground under your shoulders. Keep your body in a flat line from your shoulders all the way to your heels. You should not have your hips up in the air. As you lower your body

toward the floor, try to create a ninety-degree angle from the floor, to your elbows, to your shoulders, and then press off the ground. The entire time you're doing this exercise, remember to try to keep your body as flat as you can. Thinking about squeezing your abdominal muscles together will also help with this. If this exercise gets really tough, you can put your knees on the ground, but focus on all the tips listed above.

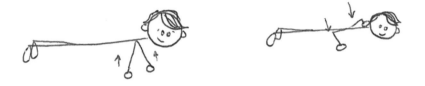

- **Squats:** Start by standing straight up with your feet shoulder width apart. Lower your body toward the floor while focusing on keeping your knees from going in front of your toes but rather, staying over your heels. As you lower yourself, imagine that you're sitting in a chair with your butt back, and keep your chin up and your back as flat as possible. Try to create a ninety-degree angle from the floor, to your knees, to your butt. Once you get to that ninety-degree angle, press off the ground with your heels, and stand back up to your starting position.

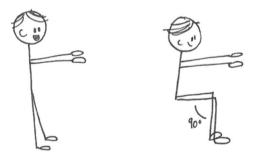

- **Sit-ups:** Lie on the ground with your butt on the floor, back flat on the ground, feet on the floor in front of you, and knees bent. Your feet will be approximately eight to twelve inches apart on the ground in front of you. Cross your arms on your chest, focus on keeping your chin back, and pick a spot to stare at ahead of you. Raise your upper body as high as you can, trying to get your chest to your knees, and then lower yourself back down. Try to remember you are pulling your body up with your abdominal muscles, so focus on tightening those and keeping your back flat.

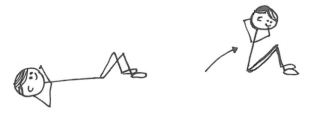

- **Lunges:** Start by standing straight up, with your hands on your hips and your feet right next to each other. Step out really far away from your body with one foot, and with your other leg, bend your knee so that it is within a few inches of the ground. Keep your back as straight as possible, and try not to lean forward as you take your step. Make sure your front knee does not go past your toes, but rather, stays over your heels. When you have your foot planted and away from your body, it is time to bring it back to your starting position by picking that foot up off the ground, pushing back, and standing straight up. Your feet should never drag on the ground during this exercise.

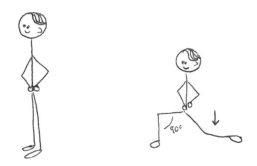

- **Jumping jacks:** Start by standing straight up, with your feet together and your hands at your side. At the same time, raise your hands together above your head and spread both of your feet apart, past the width of your shoulders. Once you get into this position, bring your hands back down to your side in a circular motion and move your feet back together. Rather than stepping with your feet, you should be doing a hop.

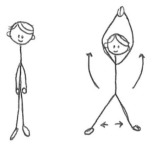

Again, we only recommend this type of regimented exercise for older children who have a legitimate interest in working out. Please don't ever force your child to workout, as it will only backfire. That being said, younger children enjoy mimicking parents and older siblings and may join in, which is fine. The whole idea here is to find a way to make it fun, so they don't even know they're exercising at all.

Adding these exercises will really test your strength and endurance. This, along with regular activity, can make getting healthier fun and make all the difference in the world.

An added benefit of exercise, and one that is little talked about, is that it makes your child feel empowered.

9

Feeling Safe in an Unsafe World

Being overweight can be frustrating and discouraging, and can lead to a cascade of negative feelings and emotions. We all know that. And at the same time, the negative feelings can also trigger emotional eating, which leads to further weight gain. It's a vicious cycle that many of us have lived through and that your child may very well be dealing with right now.

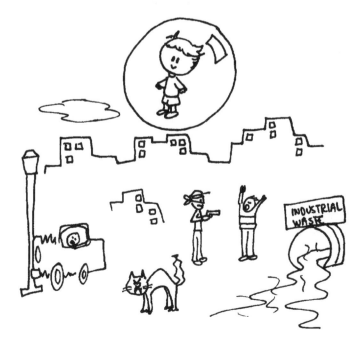

One study found that over half of clinically obese adolescents have problems with their emotional and psychosocial functioning, and these problems were significantly greater among the obese than among a normal-weight adolescent group.[1] Researchers have also examined the role of anxiety, depression, and emotional eating in overweight children and found that "individuals may lose control over their eating behavior and start to binge eat because they believe it provides distraction and comfort from painful negative emotions."[2] The problem is that after they eat, the feelings are still there.

Overweight Hispanic youth are more than twice as likely to experience mental health problems as their normal-weight counterparts, emphasizing the need for further treatment among this group.[3] There are many social and economic factors that contribute to obesity, and there are many ways that these factors can interrelate. Nonetheless, they all have an emotional component.

As important as it is to take into account the emotional life of obese individuals, it's equally important to be aware that emotions can trigger weight gain in the first place, as well as maintain or perpetuate the condition. So while feelings like depression and low self-esteem can be a *result* of obesity, what you may not be aware of is that these chronic stressors can trigger hormone responses that can *cause* obesity.

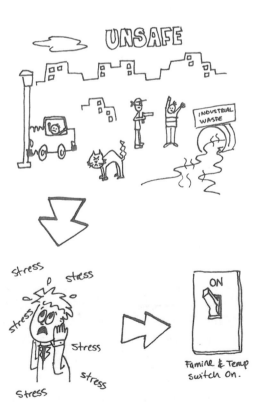

Emotional stresses are basically telling our children's bodies, that for whatever reason, they are not in a safe situation. And in the same way that famine or a long winter equals *unsafe*, causing their bodies to store more fat and gain weight, certain emotional stresses in some children will also mean *unsafe*, triggering the same FAT switch response. This feeling of being unsafe might not be immediately obvious to parents, or even the child, but that doesn't mean that it isn't there.

A local paper interviewed one of Dr. Patricia's patients after he lost close to 100 pounds. He told the reporter that he now felt like if a bad guy chased him, he could get away.

Until that point, Dr. Patricia never realized how vulnerable a 295-pound boy could feel. And while in this child's case, losing weight made him feel safer, unfortunately, for many children it's the exact opposite. Being heavier can make them feel safer.

Jon once worked with a woman who was sexually abused as a child by a female baby-sitter. This went on for three years, and the whole time she was being abused, she kept gaining weight, until the baby-sitter was no longer interested in her. In this extreme example, the weight actually did protect her. Unfortunately, this woman has now been struggling with obesity for thirty years. It's as if her body made an indelible association between being fat and being safe. Anytime she ever lost a little bit of weight, she started to feel unsafe again and started eating uncontrollably. She saw it as "self-sabotage," but the reality was that, given her history, as far as her body was concerned, the fat gain was more like "self-preservation." It wasn't until she dealt with the actual trauma that she had suffered as a child that she was finally able to let go of the weight once and for all.

One study, which looked at adverse childhood experiences (ACEs) in over seventeen thousand cases, found a statistically significant correlation between childhood trauma and health problems later in life. In other words, if a child experiences a negative, traumatic event, as an adult they are much more likely to experience health problems, such as heart disease, cancer, depression, chronic fatigue, and obesity.[4]

Emotional trauma, past or present, can lead to stress and weight gain, so the emotional threat doesn't have to be clear and present. The threat doesn't even have to be real, as a body can respond to either real or *perceived* danger by gaining weight.[5,6]

Regardless of whether or not a danger, threat, or stress is real from an outsider's perspective, we always need to err on the side of caution when dealing with our children's emotional lives. If the threat is real to *them*, then their bodies will respond accordingly. The dangers, threats, and stresses that humans experience in simpler societies and cultures are nothing like the stresses of the modern-day world.

Our children are not naturally suited to a life bombarded with packed schedules, hurried mealtimes, violent television shows and video games, and social media overload. They're absolutely not designed to cope well with mental and emotional stresses like parental relationship problems, financial troubles, chronic health problems, and broken families. Some children react to family breakups by becoming delinquents, while others become withdrawn or indifferent. And still others keep the stress inside themselves and gain weight.[7]

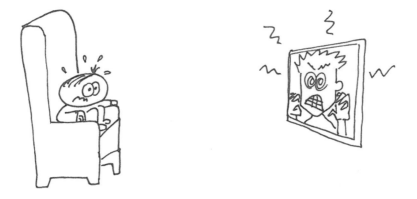

Children are also particularly ill-equipped to deal with the stresses that result from trying to live up to the false ideals, especially the false body ideals, portrayed in the media. As adults, these images can often be successful at skewing our value systems and selling us goods. If adults struggle with them, how much more do you think children struggle with or succumb to them when their capacity for analysis and criticism is so much less well developed? Significant associations have been found to support a direct relationship between television viewing and violence in youth.[8] Specifically, longitudinal studies have found associations between the time spent watching television during adolescence and the likelihood of aggressive acts toward others later in life.[9]

Some would consider media exposure and influence as a relatively small problem when compared with some of the other stresses that can traumatize children. These include:

- **A culture of violence:** This culture can be real, as in the reality of gang gunfights in the streets of a neighborhood, but it can also be virtual, like exposing kids to violent video games, television, movies, or even the violence in television news. After all, our bodies were never designed to respond to *depictions* of violence, only to real-life threats. Your body will still respond to this depicted violence as if it's just next door. It will become a chronic stress because you can't get away from it, unless you make a conscious effort to distance yourself from it. If it's real violence, you might have to move your family away physically, like moving away from your neighborhood if you can. If this isn't an option, you might have to create emotional distance by training yourself to ignore it. If it's virtual violence, you always have the option of turning off the games or television your kids are watching. Unfortunately, children aren't as good at switching off as adults are, which is why, as the guardians of their emotional lives, we have to take charge and do the switching off for them.

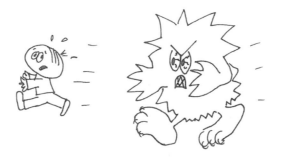

- **An environment of abuse:** Abuse takes many forms. It can be mental, emotional, physical, or sexual. We know of cases in which kids in a sexual abuse situation became obese in order to become unattractive to their abuser and then maintained that obesity into adulthood. Abuse doesn't necessarily have to be direct either. Drug abuse is a whole other level of trauma and again, it doesn't have to be direct. It's traumatizing to be the child of a drug addict or alcoholic, especially a violent one. Children may gain weight to cushion against the blows of an abusive relative or family member or use food to fill a void of love.
- **Bullying:** Although we could classify bullying as a form of abuse, we really must treat it as a separate issue. We discussed classic bullying at school in chapter 5, with tips for parents to help their children. Unfortunately, as we've seen, bullying doesn't necessarily only come from other children who might not know better, but also from adults, who ought to know better. Parents, family members, doctors, teachers, and coaches can shame children through comments in a misguided effort to help or "inspire" them, as if obese children need motivation. No one needs this kind of motivation.

Attempting to shame children through verbal, psychological, and emotional abuse is about as enlightened as attempting to cure asthma by shouting at a kid while he or she is having an attack. Bullying, if anything, is only going to make obese children want to shield themselves with more weight and turn to food as a refuge to fill their emotional void.[10]

Most children and teens want the respect of their peers. For overweight kids, this is often the one thing that they *don't* get. Bullying is something that overweight children almost always experience.[11] The thing about bullying is that it can show up in really subtle and often unintentional ways. For example, there's nothing more disheartening or dispiriting when you're overweight than wearing clothes that don't fit. They're too tight, they're unflattering, and they're uncomfortable. They constantly remind you of your weight problem. This is often part of the general humiliation associated with being an overweight kid. School uniforms are particularly problematic because they're mass-produced in a way that assumes thinness. With school uniforms, you might have to campaign for bigger sizes. In the wider commercial world, where there is more choice, the goal is to keep potential humiliation to a minimum.

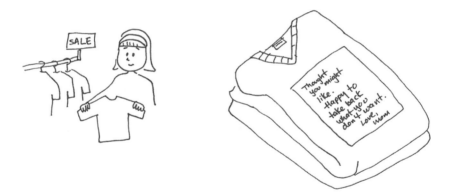

We suggest buying clothes at a regular store that carries larger sizes, or if there's one available, buy at a store that specializes in plus-size clothing. These stores are usually great because they're stocked with clothing that's especially designed to look flattering on larger bodies, and they do things with a bit more thought and sensitivity toward this market than they otherwise might. Another alternative is to purchase from plus-size stores' catalogs, so that your kids can make clothing choices without the potential embarrassment of going to a store dedicated to larger sizes.

- **A situation of loss:** The death of a parent, sibling, or other family member is extremely traumatic. We even know of cases in which a parent put on the weight equivalent of their dead child. It's equally possible for this to happen to a surviving sibling, out of sympathy or neglect. Divorce is another major, stressful life change associated with loss: loss of relationship, loss of stability, and loss of the way things used to be. Such losses are sometimes dealt with through weight gain. A families' deportation, or threat of deportation, from the country where they are living, can also be the cause of major chronic stress.

- **A situation of neglect:** Neglect is the lack of attention to the needs that must be met in order for us to stay healthy and feel safe. However, while adults are, almost by definition, people who can take responsibility and have the power to take care of their own needs, children are dependent on adults to meet their needs. Other chronic lacks of the modern world include poverty—a general lack of money for basic needs—and unemployment, which is a major factor in poverty. Although, as many of the working poor know, you don't have to be unemployed to be experiencing major financial stress.

How you deal with all these stresses depends on your means and the level of seriousness of the trauma. It's unlikely that you'll be able to deal with serious abuse issues like alcoholism or sexual abuse without some form of professional intervention, so if you know, or even suspect, that your child might be in a

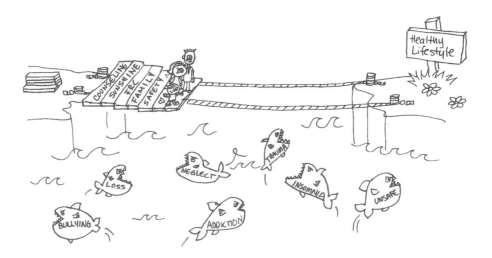

situation of abuse, we'd advise getting professional help. There are also many different types of therapy and services available to help both adults and children deal with emotional stress. Many communities have support organizations for families in need. Work with your pediatrician or family practice doctor for referrals. If you have access to the Internet, feel free to access our website online for a listing of these resources.

10

Using the Mind-Body Connection to Improve Emotional Health

In order to create a truly effective and sustainable approach to health and fitness for our children, we need to involve both the mind and the body. We know that stress and negative emotions can cause children to gain weight.[1,2,3] So we need tools for addressing these issues. We need tools for helping our children solve emotional problems, cope with painful experiences, and resolve past traumas. If you can help your child develop effective strategies for dealing with these daily stresses, you'll also be giving them an invaluable, lifelong skill. And if weight is an issue, it will help with it as well.

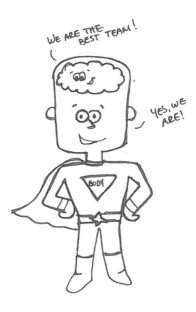

If there's a place that we can say that the basic emotions "live," it's the limbic region of the brain. If there's a place that we can call the "seat of fear and emotion," it's in an almond-sized area of the limbic system called the *amygdala*. Conditions such as anxiety, autism, depression, PTSD, and phobias are suspected to be linked to the abnormal functioning of the amygdala.[4]

One really important thing to realize is that when something stimulates the amygdala, when something evokes certain fearful emotions, your brain doesn't care where that stimulation comes from. That's why you feel things regardless of whether they come from something in the outside world or are purely the result of something that you dream, imagine, or even talk yourself into. That's why movies, music, and books can evoke feelings, like excitement or fear, just as effectively as if you were in a real fun or dangerous situation. It's why you probably shouldn't read horror stories before you go to bed.

The amygdala is the seat of negative emotions, such as fear, and every time something stimulates the amygdala, it causes a stress response that elevates the levels of the stress hormone *cortisol*.[5] As cortisol builds up, it becomes easier to experience more stress, because in a state of high stress, even the wiring in your brain changes. When that happens, you get caught up in a repetitive pattern of stress building on stress. Cortisol also leads to weight gain. It's a vicious cycle that can quickly lead to obesity and compromised health. So how do you break the cycle of stress building on stress?

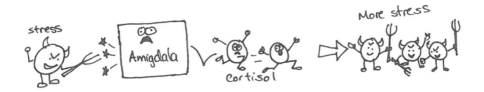

We have already spoken about how exercise, better communication, sleep, and the creation of healthy relationships with food can be beneficial ways of managing stress. Another powerful tool to help deal with stress is meditation.

A lot of people hear the word *meditation*, and they think that it's something complicated or religious or weird, but it really isn't any of these things at all. Meditation is simply a state of mind in which you are calm, relaxed, and feel safe and at peace, but you are still awake and softly alert. Even brainwave patterns change. Many people describe this state as a feeling of "presence" or of being "in the moment." There are many ways to achieve this state. Sometimes it's as simple as sitting still with your eyes half-closed and breathing deeply, slowly, and steadily, softly concentrating on your breathing. We'll outline a method of getting into a meditative state in the coming pages, but for now, just understand that it's a very nice feeling, one that's perfectly safe and not at all mysterious or spooky. The benefits of meditation are many and include:

- Feelings of relaxation and quiet
- Slowing of the heart rate

- Lowering of blood pressure
- Calming of the nerves
- A general feeling of well-being

Studies have also shown that meditation lowers cortisol levels and inhibits signals to the amygdala.[6] Several studies have also been conducted having obese individuals practice meditation. The results show that when obese participants practiced mindfully based and focused eating, significant changes occurred in weight, eating behavior, and stress.[7] In addition, mindfulness and meditation were found to be effective in weight management because they reconnect you to internal signs, and they help you to improve self-regulation.[8]

Take the case of the purported world's happiest man, French Buddhist monk and advisor to the Dalai Lama, Matthieu Ricard. Neuroscientist Richard Davison has measured the sixty-six-year-old's brain waves and discovered that after having practiced meditation for forty years, when Matthieu meditates specifically on compassion, he generates levels of gamma waves "never reported before in the neuroscience literature."[9]

"The scans also showed excessive activity in his brain's left prefrontal cortex compared to its right counterpart, giving him an abnormally large capacity for happiness and a reduced propensity towards negativity, researchers believe." Furthermore, Davison maintains that "it shows that meditation is not just blissing out under a mango tree but it completely changes your brain and therefore changes what you are."[10]

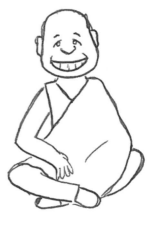

If meditation can produce the world's happiest man, it might make a big difference to your life and to the lives of your children. And you don't have to wait forty years to gain the benefits.[11] Meditation can be guided or unguided. In unguided meditation, you just get into a relaxed, alert state and let your thoughts drift wherever they will, while you calmly observe those thoughts without commentary or judgment, rather like a pleasant dream.

In guided meditation, you're either listening to a voice that provides you with instructions, like is sometimes done in yoga classes, or you are steering your own thoughts in a particular direction for a particular purpose. Guided meditation involves actively imagining things.

Visualization is a form of guided meditation. Now, although visualization implies seeing things with your mind's eye or steering your thoughts through visual imagery, in fact visualization can also mean creating feelings too. You create a peaceful scene, for example, by imagining sitting on a beach. But you don't have to just see the beach with your mind's eye and confine yourself to seeing how the waves look as they crash on the shore or how the sun looks in the blue sky. You're free to use your mind's ear to hear the sound of the wind and the waves and the cries of seagulls. You can smell the air with your mind's nose. You can taste the salt with your mind's tongue and feel the sand and sunlight with your mind's skin. This might take some practice, but it's worth trying and persisting to get to a place where you can use all your senses, as it makes visualizations more powerful.

Because visualization is a form of meditation, simply getting into a meditative or visualization state will rewire your brain circuitry and orient it more toward pleasure and relaxation, and away from stress and fear.[12] In essence, you're rewiring your brain chemistry so you can experience fitness, happiness, and success. The great thing about visualization is that if you do it in the morning, the benefits of rewiring your brain to be in a calm, relaxed, but alert state will last the whole day.[13] But visualization is so much more than just a way to create a happy, peaceful place in your head, because at a neurological level the mind can't distinguish between a real or imagined state, it treats visualization as being as real as anything else we might experience.

Visualization is a tremendously powerful tool for communicating with your body and establishing and reinforcing the link between guided thoughts and real changes that can occur in your body. In fact, studies have shown that Olympic athletes can visualize training and winning at their sports while sit-

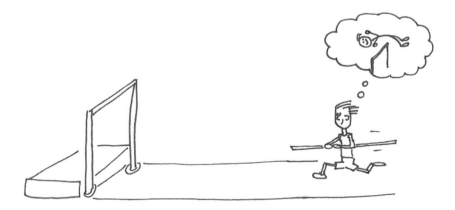

ting or lying down, and their bodies will respond with the same coordinated sequence of nerves firing and muscles moving, as if they were actually in the field.[14] But it gets better.

Visualization can be a very powerful tool to help you achieve your goals. It's like being able to rehearse the necessary thoughts, feelings, actions, scenarios, and changes that you need for success in the comfort and safety of your own space, as often as you want. You don't even have to work out all the details of the path to success either. It's incredibly helpful to visualize the end result as clearly as you can, and then let the details take care of themselves. Motivational experts, like Louise Hay, Deepak Chopra, Wayne Dyer, Tony Robbins, and Oprah Winfrey, and athletes, like Michael Jordan, Tiger Woods, and Carl Lewis, all credit visualization for their success. What works for them can work for you, your family, and your children.

Benefits of Visualization

- Improves schoolwork and raises exam scores
- Improves performance in recreational games or sports
- Helps you conquer addictions like alcoholism or smoking
- Helps you overcome health problems, recover from procedures, and cures psychological and medical conditions
- And most importantly for our purposes, it helps you create a healthy lifestyle.[15]

Jon credits the practice of visualization with not only solving his own weight issues, but with helping tens of thousands of people all over the world lose weight and keep it off in an easy and sustainable way. Helping our minds and bodies feel calm, safe, protected, and unstressed is essential to weight loss. Thus, helping your kids visualize themselves as being safe, secure, and protected sends their bodies an incredibly powerful message that says it's okay to lose their excess fat.

Children, especially young children, are famously unable to distinguish between imagination and reality, which is an incredible advantage for visualization. Children are excellent natural visualizers, and they benefit dramatically from visualization.[16,17] Jon frequently hears from parents how effective visualization has been for their kids in losing weight. One of the greatest gifts that you can give your kids is an introduction to visualization and, though anyone can gain its benefits at any time, the earlier they start, the better.

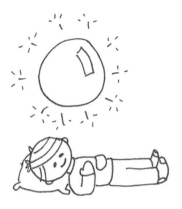

Visualization is like a musical instrument. The more you practice it, the better you get and the more rewarding the results will be. So if you introduce the habit of daily visualization to a child, he or she will soon learn to master the technique and can then apply it, not only to health and fitness, but also to any area of life he or she wishes to excel in. It's a simple, cheap, pleasurable, and extremely effective lifelong tool for helping children achieve their goals. It's a gift that keeps on giving.

How to Visualize

The key to successful visualization is to get your kids into a relaxed state. When children are properly relaxed, they go into what scientists call the *alpha* and *theta* brainwave states. In these states, children are calmer, clearer, more focused, and their thought processes are actually more powerful. In these states, accelerated learning can take place, so habits can be made, changed, or broken very quickly, and your children can forge new habits, associations, and desired outcomes *instantly*.[18]

To get your kids into these states, use guided imagery. Consciousness researchers have discovered that if you focus on a particular part of the body, it will relax. So first, get your kids to lie down on a bed or on a couch and make sure they're comfortable. Then, the next step is to walk your child through the relaxation process. There are several ways you can do this. One way is to ask your child to imagine a ball of white light inside her body, maybe the size of a tennis ball. This will engage her visual imagination.

The next step is to tell her to imagine the ball of white light traveling to different parts of her body. Get her to take her time. Start at the toes and end at the head. Suggest to her that wherever the ball of light touches, that part of the body will become relaxed. Once the light has finished its journey through the body, it can then rest around the child's navel. At this point, your child should be relaxed and calm, but still alert. Now you can start making suggestions to your child as to what to visualize.

You're guiding this process, and you're responsible for what you say, so it's important to say things in the right way. Using positive statements and positive language is really important. To understand why, try this. Close your eyes and say to yourself, "I hate chocolate cake." What happens? The moment you hear "chocolate cake," you form some sort of image of chocolate cake, and you start salivating because your body is responding to that image. So you want to change your language so that the focus is on what you want, not what you don't want or what you want to exclude. What you need to do instead is to see yourself being vital and healthy. This principle applies to what you're going to suggest to your child.

Saying "See yourself, strong and healthy, at the park climbing, jumping, running around, and playing" is a much more powerful and effective statement than suggesting that "You hate being inactive." Also, specific statements about food might violate the proper psychology of feeding your child, and we recommend avoiding them altogether when doing visualization. So when doing visualization, it's best not to mention food, but instead to emphasize other aspects of being active or engaging in a healthy lifestyle.

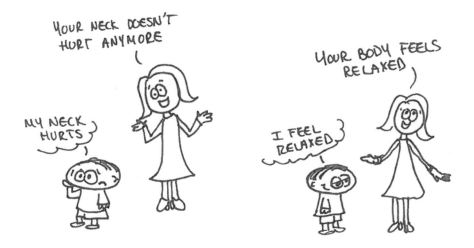

However, it's fine to use the imagery of food in a symbolic way. To find how this works, see the way we use the imagery of berries in the magic-carpet-ride visualization below.

Then there are also passive statements versus active statements. There are two ways of phrasing statements that you should make to your child: indirect and direct. Use these different styles for different reasons.

Here's an example of an indirect statement: "You might find that you'll start to enjoy your active, healthy body." Here's an example of a direct statement: "You love playing outdoors with your friends."

At the beginning of a visualization session, children's conscious minds are more active and more likely to fight a positive statement that they don't agree with. So at the beginning of a session, it's more helpful to use language like, "You might . . ." or "It's possible that . . ." or "Perhaps . . ."

But the longer you're in a session, the deeper children will be into the alpha or theta state. The conscious mind takes a holiday, so it won't be there to get in the way of your suggestions. You'll know that your child is deeply into a meditative or visualization state when they stop fidgeting, and their breathing is calm and regular. And if they are really deep into the state, their eyelashes will flutter because their eyes are moving rapidly under their lids, just like they do when they're dreaming during REM sleep. The difference here is that they're not asleep; their state of consciousness is actually closer to those dreamy, twilight moments just before you fall asleep. It's in this state that they will receive most of the positive change that you're guiding them to.

We recommend that you practice these visualizations every night with your kids. We find that during visualizations, children respond best to images or stories of journeys. Creating your own visualizations for your children and getting into this state requires some persistence and practice on both your parts. To make it easier, here are a couple of examples for different age groups that incorporate the principles that we've just talked about (see also, appendix I, Visualizations, for additional examples).

The Magic Carpet Ride

This visualization is geared toward early school-aged kids:

Tonight we're going to go on a magic carpet ride. So as you're lying down, take a deep breath in, release a deep breath out, and relax. Let everything go. And as you're lying there in your bed, imagine that there's a cuddly, lovable monkey next to you, and she's loving, supportive, and protective—all she wants is to play with you, love you, and protect you.

As she's sitting there next to you on the bed, I'd like you to imagine that the bed becomes a magic carpet, and you go flying up in the air. The monkey is protecting you all the way, and it's so much fun. You go up into the sky, and as you're flying on this magic carpet, it feels so fun and so easy and so relaxed. You can see the whole world and the sun from where you are.

You and the monkey are flying to a beautiful, magical palace. And as she's flying with you, it feels so relaxing—you can feel your whole body relaxing. You start letting go. You can feel your legs relaxing, your ribs relaxing, and your eyelids relaxing as you lie on this beautiful magic carpet with this cuddly, loving monkey. You can feel your neck relaxing and your head relaxing and your arms relaxing. It feels so good. You're flying around, and you're way up in the sky. You can see the whole world from up there. You feel safe and protected, and at the same time, it's so much fun.

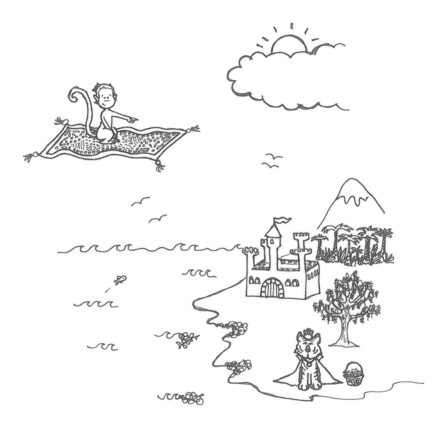

The farther you fly, the more relaxed and the happier you feel. All your cares go away. They just melt away, and you feel calm, happy, safe, protected, and nurtured. And as you're flying on this magic carpet, you can see in the distance a beautiful palace resting above the clouds, where the monkey's taking you. And she says, "I'm taking you to my magic palace. This is my home, and you can meet the most magic tiger in the whole world."

So she takes you to this palace. When the magic carpet gently lands, she takes your hand and helps you off. The two of you walk hand in hand up the stairs, one step at a time, to this beautiful palace, with its tall ceilings, beautiful arches, stones, diamonds, and gold. There are people there that help you; guards and servants salute you as you walk up the stairs with this magic monkey.

As you're walking, you see that there's a tiger there to greet you, and he has the most loving, beautiful eyes. He's a kind tiger. He's a wise tiger, and he's a powerful tiger. You walk up to the top of the stairs with your monkey. She introduces you and says, "This is the most magic tiger in the whole world. He can do anything. He can make anything happen." And he smiles at you and says, "Today, I'm going to give you some special blessings to make you strong, happy, healthy, and successful in every area of your life."

He has a plate of delicious berries that he picked from his garden, and he says to you, "These are magic berries. They are very powerful, and each one has a special purpose." He hands you one, and you taste it, and it's so delicious and nutritious. You can feel your body being nourished, and he says, "That berry is to make you feel safe and loved and strong and confident." You eat the berry, and you feel safe and loved and strong and confident.

Then he gives you another berry and says, "This berry is to make you feel fit and strong and super healthy." You eat the berry, and instantly you feel your body getting stronger and healthier. And in an instant, you can see yourself feeling strong, energized, fast, and happy.

He gives you another berry and says, "This berry is so that you'll love jumping, climbing, and playing games with your friends more than anything in the world." He gives you that berry, and you eat it, and you see yourself running as fast as the wind. You can see yourself playing sports with your friends, running, climbing, skipping, and jumping, and excelling in any sport or game that you're playing and being truly, truly happy. You just love to run like the wind. It's pure joy. It's so much fun to move your body, and you love the way your body feels. You love to run and move and climb and play. It's so much fun. And you love playing with your friends, and they're having fun too. Everybody's having a great time. You're chasing, running, jumping, climbing, and skipping, and it feels so good.

He gives you another berry and says, "This berry is so that you'll love the joy of learning, and you'll easily learn everything that you want to learn at school, and learning will be fun and enjoyable." And you eat that berry, and you can see yourself in school really loving to learn new things. It's so easy and effortless. You just learn all the things at school so easily, and you're smiling, and you're raising your hand. You might even be the first one to raise your hand, and you've got the answer, things make sense to you, and you're so happy. Learning is so easy and effortless for you.

He gives you one last berry and says, "This berry is so that you will love the joy of sleeping, and you will easily fall deeply asleep. You will dream happy dreams, and you will wake up in the morning feeling rested. You will wake up calm and comfortable, but with the strength and energy to move mountains." Through your deep, long sleep everything seems easy and effortless. You feel powerful, strong, healthy, and rested, and the world is yours.

Then he gives you a special gold medallion and says, "This medallion will tie everything together. With this medallion, you will be happy, healthy, strong, and will love the joy of movement, and it will be so easy and effortless for you to learn and to sleep soundly, waking up feeling fresh and powerful." And you put this medallion, this beautiful gold medallion, around you, and in an instant, you see yourself at school the next day. You see yourself running like the wind and raising your hand in class and getting the answer right. You see your body getting stronger, healthier, and happier, and you're smiling. You're beaming a happy smile all day. And you are fresh after a good night's sleep, and it's the most beautiful, enjoyable day that you've ever had in your whole life.

You thank this special, magic tiger, and you and your friendly guide, the monkey, go hand in hand down the steps, one by one. Farther and farther down, one step at a time, back to the magic carpet. And as you go farther and farther down, one step at a time, to your magic carpet, you feel so relaxed, so happy. You know, beyond a shadow of a doubt, that something has changed in you, that your body now feels safe, healthy, and happy, that your body wants to run like the wind and play, that your mind is focused, that it's so easy to learn, and that you can see yourself beaming a smile all day long after a refreshing sleep. And as you go farther and farther down, one step at a time, and reach your magic carpet, you and your monkey get on your magic carpet, and you easily and effortlessly drift back into the sky, back over the clouds, passing over oceans and land, until you very gently and effortlessly land back in your bed, where you finally allow yourself to drift off into a deep, deep sleep.

Bedtime

The time before bed is the best time to instill new ways of looking at the world, and it's an especially powerful time for young children. With that in mind, you can further reinforce the principles of visualization with some powerful storytelling. It is also a great help with reading, vocabulary, focus, and most importantly, bonding.[19] Even making a habit of a nightly prayer or blessing, depending on your religious beliefs, can be a powerful tool to bond and get perspective before going to bed.

Bedtime Stories for Children Five Years Old and Younger

These tales promote bonding and positive messages. Dr. Patricia has a collection of stories she reads to her daughter as she tucks her in at night. She wrote *The Dreaming Tree* and *There are so Many Kisses* herself, and there's nothing stopping you from writing your own stories for your children (see also, appendix I, Visualizations). We also recommend *Goodnight Moon* by Margaret Wise Brown, *Ruby Valentine* by Laurie B. Friedman, *The Night I Followed the Dog* by Nina Laden, *Stella Luna* by Janell Cannon, and *A Magical Day with Matisse* by Julie Merberg and Suzanne Bober.

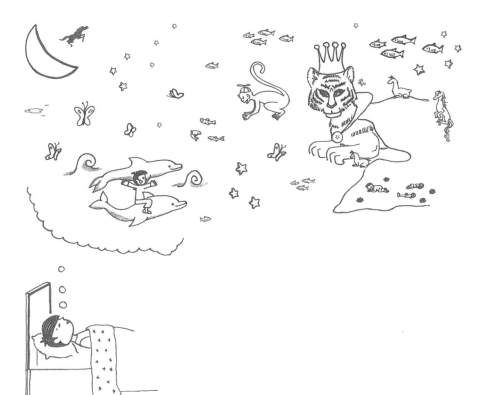

The Dreaming Tree

Under a great and brilliant moon,
A Dreaming Tree outside your room,
Makes rainbows bright that never fade,
While children sleep beneath its shade,
It speaks in silent whispers too,
That somehow turn to dreams in you.
Dreams that start with butterflies,
Who sing sweet gentle lullabies,
And carry you on cotton wings,
To worlds made bright with magic things,
Flying horses, singing llamas,
Fish that swim in your pajamas,
Spiders spinning webs of gold,
And with their threads new dreams are told,
Dreams that tell you that you're free
To be whatever you will be
The branches of the tree reach high,
To stroke the black and silky sky,
And on the branches flowers bloom,
That glow with starlight from the moon,
And on the twigs the leaves unfurl
And stretch until they then uncurl
Each leaf a page of recollections,
Taking you to new directions,
You'll climb, you'll dance, you'll fly, you'll glide,
You'll shape those dreams you keep inside,
You'll play with life, you'll gather stuff,
You'll gather 'till you have enough,
And then you'll share your odds and ends,
With present, past and future friends,
All this and more, such wondrous joys
For little girls and little boys
Tucked in their beds, all safe and sound,
All safe to dream their dreams unbound,
And as the clock does quietly tick,
There's time for one last secret trick,

Let every dream, your heart ignite,
And reach, reach, for the stars tonight.
Good night . . .

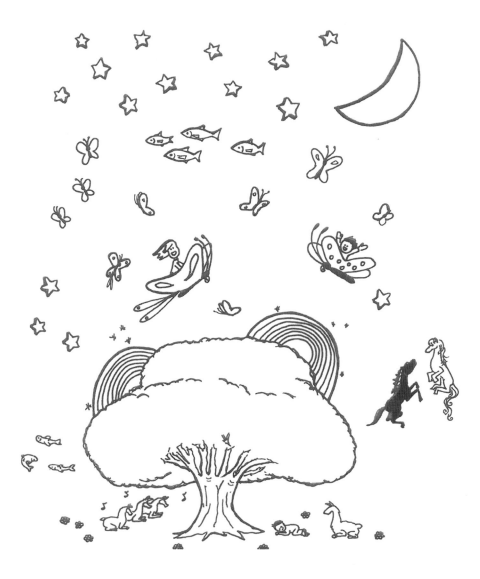

As in so many other cases, visualization and storytelling are techniques for which practice makes perfect. The more you practice visualization with your kids, the better you'll get. And when your kids get more confident, they can create their own visualizations. As you start seeing the results, confidence will grow too.

We all have limitations, often self-imposed, that can interfere with our ability to be healthy. It is really important that you examine what these limitations might be. It's important to empower yourself by becoming as mentally, emotionally and physically healthy as you can. When you're coming from your own place of power, you become an example of health for your children. Jon provides visualizations for parents too, which may be a good start. Find ways to overcome the barriers in your own life, so you can create positive changes in all aspects of your children's environment without the added obstacle of being at war with yourself too.

Visit TheGabrielMethod.com/FitKids for more guided visualizations and DrRibasHealthClub.org/FitKids for more children's bedtime stories.

11

Improve Yourself, Improve Your Child's Health

One of the best things you can do to help improve your child's health and fitness is to heal yourself. In the movie *Dead Poets Society*, the teacher (played by Robin Williams) asks his students to stand on their desks in order to look at the classroom from a different perspective. This model has been a great source of inspiration for Dr. Patricia when coming upon an obstacle she needs to get past. Sometimes, stepping back and reflecting to see if there is a better way to approach the problem is the most effective way to accomplish things.

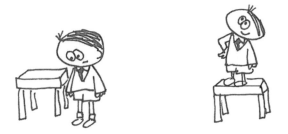

Either consciously or unconsciously, our children are modeling themselves after us—our actions, beliefs, attitudes, feelings, ideas, world, and relationships are all being taken in, absorbed, and modeled by our children. Children eat more vegetables if their moms eat more vegetables. Studies have found that in role-playing scenarios, preschool children will mimic their parents' food choices.[1] The healthier *we* are as individuals, the healthier our children will be.

Most people, when trying to deal with an overweight child, get frustrated because they're asking themselves: How do I get Johnny to behave? How do I get Janey to change? How do I get them to eat less, get some discipline, exercise more, and control their food cravings? In other words, the focus is always on how to *control* or *change* the child, usually through influence, and when that fails, then through coercion and threats.

We'd like to suggest that it's possible that you'll have much more control and be much more effective in changing the situation if you focus attention on changing yourself and some of your own patterns first.

Maternal stress has been shown to strongly influence a child's development.[2,3] The happier, more empowered, and complete you are as a person, the more those feelings will positively influence your children.

First, you need to examine your own upbringing and issues around food— its selection, preparation, and eating.

1. What were the feeding dynamics at your house when you were growing up?
2. Did you eat to deal with your emotions? Do you now? (Children can see this.)
3. Did you have to clean your plate?
4. Were you overweight as a child?
5. Were you a picky eater?
6. Were you a pleaser?
7. Were your food preferences labeled? ("She is a good eater," or "He is a bad eater.")
8. Were you labeled as a child? ("She hates vegetables," or "He never eats apples.")
9. Did you eat to live or live to eat?

Next, examine how you eat and cook now. Obviously, your attitude toward food and cooking depends on context. Sometimes you might be feeling creative in the kitchen; other times you might feel that if you have to cook one more meal for your family, you'll go insane. Sometimes you'll be feeling adventurous, and you'll want to try new things; other times you'll be happy to stick to your old favorites. Everyone goes through phases with food and cooking, loving it or hating it and everything in between. Some people are generally more conservative with food than others, while others are always trying something new. Everyone has their own food preferences.

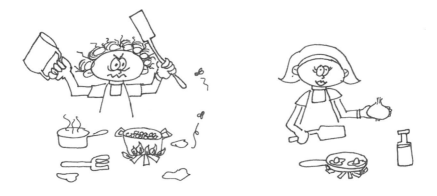

Your children might be born with certain food preferences, which might not be the same as yours. But as we know, preferences can be acquired too. What's certain is that it's much harder to get kids enthusiastic at mealtimes, especially about healthy food, if they're growing up in a household where the main food preparer hates cooking and even manages to burn water. If you can't find the energy to change your negative attitudes about food or cooking, when possible, it might be a good idea to find someone else to do the cooking, like a grandmother, aunt, uncle, or friend. Also, keep in mind that you will likely not be truly cooking as much if you adopt these principles and recipes. You'll be mostly making salads, chopping fruits and vegetables, and throwing some ingredients into a blender. There may be fewer pots and pans to clean up as you incorporate these healthy, not overcooked, and not overprepared foods into your life.

The following are some questions you might ask yourself while you ponder your attitudes about food, dieting, cooking, exercise, stress, and weight. The better you understand where you are coming from, the easier you can shift your perspectives (like standing on the desk):

- **What are your issues with and attitudes toward junk food?** Sometimes kids acquire a junk food preference from their parents. If you think that junk food is okay or that it's a treat, then your kids will learn that from you, and they'll think of junk food as a reward for being good. This is not at all the attitude that we'd like children to have, particularly if they have weight issues. And it's frankly impossible to teach your kids that junk food is not fun if you think that it is. Through your own experiences, you will need to find that healthy foods can be a fun treat, before your children will also adopt this belief. And the sooner you come to grips with this idea, the better it will be for you and your kids.

- **What are your issues with weight, diets, and calorie control?** If you've had a weight issue yourself, and you've tried diets again and again, only to experience inevitable failures over and over, then it's likely that you'll approach a new method of weight management with cynicism, pessimism, and general negativity. You'll be of two minds: half of you will already be preparing yourself for disappointment, while the other half will be hoping that *this time* it will work. It's likely that you'll pass this pessimism along to your children, however unconsciously. Although it's sometimes easier said than done, it's important to stay positive. In our experience, the best way to do this is to fully acknowledge any success that you or your kids experience and to treat any "failure" as simply a temporary setback. It also pays to be realistic. Dealing with weight issues takes time, and there are inevitable plateaus and temporary reversals. Nothing creates enthusiasm like lasting success, and that comes from weight management approaches that actually work. The "success" that comes from dieting is only an illusion. The more little successes that you and your family share—and this sort of success is always shared—the more you'll be set up for the big success of long-term, sustainable weight loss.

- **How do you feel about your body?** Do you love your body? Do you hate it? Do you accept your body? It's hard to teach your children to accept their own bodies if you're constantly subconsciously rejecting your own body or maybe even rejecting theirs. Kids have a built-in hypocrisy detector when it comes to their parents, which is why saying "Do as I say, not as I do" never really works. What works even less is saying "Feel as I say, not as I feel." Again, it's easier said than done, but you have to love your body no matter how it may look to you. It helps to know that even obesity is simply a result of your body trying to keep you safe and alive. Your body really does love you. Obesity, whatever disadvantages it has, is more of a well-intentioned error than a sign that you hate yourself or that your body hates you.

  It also helps to neither give any validity to other peoples' judgments about your body nor to compare yourself constantly to standards set by society or the mass media. Some people with the most negative and dysfunctional attitudes toward their bodies are fashion and fitness models. It might sound odd, but sometimes the easiest path to accepting your body and your child's body is simply to stop rejecting them. Find things to appreciate about your bodies. Appreciation works wonders.

- **How physically active are you?** Once again, it's hard to convincingly extol the benefits of exercise to your children if you're a confirmed couch potato. We've already said that it's not a good idea to associate activity with exercise. There are many ways to be physically engaged. Find some physical activity that you love to do, and do it. It doesn't matter if your child chooses a different activity; you simply need to model activity *in*

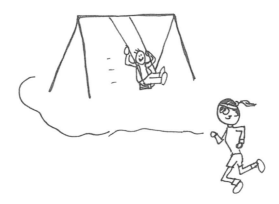

principle, because your children won't believe that movement can be fun unless you believe it yourself. Part of the problem with activity can be the way that it's sold to us. Are you ever physically active for the sheer joy of movement, or is it all just grueling workouts full of laps or reps? Children respond much better to exercise when it's fun, rather than when it's some sort of physical regime to put themselves through in order to win a sport or look a certain way.

- **How stressful is your life?** Does stress permeate your home life so that your child feels your stress through osmosis? How you deal with stress will affect how your children deal with stress, and as we know, *any* stress is a potential danger. We've already talked about how there are healthy and unhealthy ways to deal with stress. Find effective ways to deal with your own stress, and you'll be more empowered to help your children deal with the stresses that they encounter. Try to control the emotional atmosphere in the house—the last thing that your children need is stress by osmosis. If you can generate calm in yourself, you'll be creating a home environment in which it's easier for your child to find refuge from stress too.

- **How strong are the boundaries in your personal and professional relationships?** Obesity often occurs when people are trying to define a space for themselves. Sometimes obesity pushes people away; sometimes obesity protects people from attack. If you can gain the skills to establish firm boundaries, then you'll no longer need to use obesity as a way of maintaining boundaries. In turn, your children will learn how to create healthy boundaries from you, so they will be less likely to suffer from emotional weight gain.

- **Have you suffered from abusive relationships?** Do you have unresolved issues around any past abusive relationships? Are you currently involved in an abusive relationship, either personally or professionally? Is that pattern of abuse contaminating your relationship with your child?

  A child should always feel safe at home and should not be exposed to the toxicity of habitual drama or arguments. The connection between abuse and obesity is an extension of the boundary issue, because abuse always involves a violation of boundaries and the destruction of trust. Abuse can be psychological, emotional, physical, or sexual, and can exist within a workplace relationship, friendship, a marriage, between parents and their children, or with total strangers; you get the picture. Dealing with abuse is a topic beyond the scope of this book, but we're simply pointing out that you need to sort out any abuse issues and get help. Abuse that affects children, even indirectly, can cause boundary problems for a child, because any abuse means the child is *unsafe*. Until you resolve your own abusive relationships, you won't have the means to keep your children from establishing similar abusive patterns that might create stresses and negatively affect their health.

- **How safe do you think the world is?** How safe do you feel in general? Feeling unsafe, especially chronically, is a huge source of stress for many. Suffice it to say, the safer and more secure you feel, the safer and more secure your child is going to feel, because children take their safety cues from their parents. Children are profoundly affected when they see adults in a state of anxiety or fear. Fears and feelings of being unsafe can be either rational or irrational. Rational fears need to be handled with practical measures, while irrational fears often need professional help.

- **Are you engaged with life?** Are you passionate about life, or is your life full of fear and escapism in order to avoid your reality? Are you in love with life, or is it just something you have to get through? You can't truly engage with life if you are feeling unsafe, because it's impossible to be enthusiastic about life from a place of fear and trepidation. An important gift you can give your child is that feeling of engagement. No other feeling is more contagious, but you have to infect yourself with it first by satisfying your own emotional needs. It's like the advice that they give you on an airplane: in case of emergency, put *your* oxygen mask on first before you help your children put on theirs. And it's much more likely that you'll look after your own emotional needs if you love and respect yourself in the first place.

How much love and respect you give yourself has a direct bearing on how your children learn to love themselves. Every self-deprecating, self-belittling, self-devaluing statement, feeling, belief, or behavior that you create for yourself will influence the way your children feel about themselves, purely through unconscious assimilation of thought patterns. This might require a lot of work on your part, but you can't expect your family to change unless you demonstrate your own capacity to change, both for your own sake and for theirs.

Children don't come into the world knowing how to live and how to be in the world. They take their cues from you, and like it or not, you are their first and most important formative role model. You need to show them how to live through your example. Actions speak louder, longer, and more often than words, and kids will always take their cues from your actions. Your example to your children comes not only from how you act, but even more so from the thoughts, beliefs, and feelings that form the foundation of your acts.

It all really comes down to an issue of authority and credibility. Simply put, there is no greater influence that you can have or exert over your child than that of changing yourself and making yourself healthier.

We encourage you to start by adopting some of the healthy habits and suggestions in this book, like practicing meditation and visualization; reconnecting with the joy of being physically active; adding real, live, vibrant foods to your diet; getting lots of good, quality sleep; finding your passion; and most of all, practicing being patient, gentle, loving, accepting, and forgiving with yourself. Treat yourself exactly the way you would treat your child, family member, or friend whom you love and adore, and you'll be teaching your children the greatest possible lesson: self-love.

12

Home Is Where the Health Is

In order to help our children be healthy, we need to create a healthy home for them to grow and thrive in. At this point in the book, you should feel very comfortable with the fact that diets and portion control do not work and instead make children feel more stressed, more food insecure, and less happy during mealtimes. You need to control what you can—buy and serve foods rich in nutrition and make mealtimes pleasant, warm, and inviting, and then let your child self-regulate the foods you are serving. These steps can increase your child's nutritional intake, decrease junk food cravings, and decrease stress, all of which leads to sustainable health and fitness.

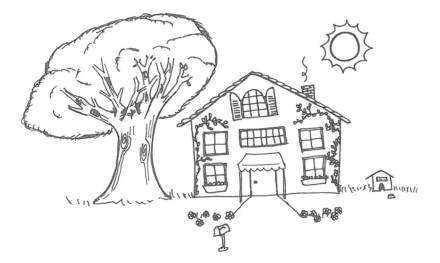

But let's also look at some of the other ways we can create health in the home. Children are intimately connected to everything that they encounter in their lives, and their most frequent, intense, important encounters and connections are with their families, especially in the early years. Healthier families generally mean healthier kids.

One good place to start is making sure your child has good access to medical, dental, and psychological services. A toothache might make a child not want to eat an apple or a carrot, and a simple tooth cleaning can have a substantial impact on health and body weight. Pathogens in periodontal disease are inflammatory and elevate the levels of inflammatory hormones that can cause weight gain.[1] So if your child hasn't had a dental checkup recently, it might be worth making an appointment.

Also, many medical problems can affect a child's mood, desire to move, and food choices. Sleep apnea, being on medications, like steroids or antidepressants, or a history of abuse or trauma could each be causing weight gain and acting as a barrier to your child's good health. Working with a healthcare professional to treat problems or eliminate treatments that are not working are great first steps.

One thing to keep in mind is that not all healthcare professionals are aware of the latest and most effective approaches to treating childhood obesity. They may come right out and say that your child needs to lose weight without realizing that your family is actually making a tremendous effort and that your child has already lost 20 pounds. This can be very demoralizing for your child. When Dr. Patricia trains fellow physicians, she tells them to always ask if the child has been losing or gaining weight lately, regardless of the child's current weight. That way, if a 300-pound child has just lost 100 pounds (an amazing accomplishment!), the child will not be lectured about still needing to lose more weight.

Right from the start, explain to your doctor or healthcare professional that you have been making positive changes, that your whole family is working hard, and that you are very proud of them. The first step in sustainable weight loss is to simply stop the progression of weight gain. Because don't forget, children are still growing, so if they continue to grow and stop gaining, they will be slimming. Following this approach, the efforts to stop the excessive gaining should be recognized as a tremendous accomplishment. So please keep this in mind and communicate to your doctor how the scale might not be the best indicator of your family's efforts.

The next step, as we spoke about in the previous chapter, is to look at your own health and stress management. If you heal yourself first, then you'll have the space, energy, and clarity you need to help your family heal. In reality, it's hard to separate your healing from your family's healing. Your self-love and self-nurturing is nourishing to everyone in your life, especially your kids. They can feel it, they will emulate it, and the entire home environment will feel more relaxed, safe, enjoyable, and harmonious.

This may not be easy for you as a parent, because you want to help your children first, but ultimately your own self-love, your own self-respect, and your own healing is absolutely critical in your mission to help your child. It's hard to draw the line, but if you tune into your needs, you'll know when it's time to take care of you. We can't emphasize strongly enough how important it is that you take the time to nurture yourself. It's not just for you; it's for your kids and your entire family.

So, if there's a major trauma from childhood that you have never (or inadequately) dealt with, or depression, stress, sleep deprivation, a dysfunctional relationship with food, or just plain exhaustion, find the help you need. In the long run, this will help your child the most.

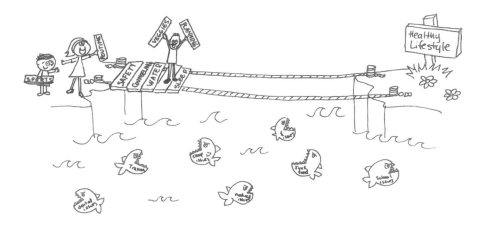

Create Solidarity through a United Front

Solidarity and consistency are so important. Parents, siblings, grandparents, and extended family members all need to understand the rules about nutrition, exercise, and healthy lifestyle choices. As families, we need to work together as much as possible. One way to achieve this is to call a family conference. Or talk to family members individually to arrive at a consensus. Attempt this on your own, but do not hesitate to seek professional help if need be. Ultimately, everyone has to be steering in the same direction.

You don't want the good work of one family member to be undermined by the counterproductive, though well intentioned (or sometimes not-so-well intentioned) acts of another. In other words, it's not okay if Grandpa is constantly smuggling in junk food. As a family, you're all in this together. It doesn't matter what shape or size each child is; there is one family plan, which will make the whole family healthier. The same approach to mind-body health and fitness will help everyone. It will help Dad's blood pressure go down; it will help an underweight or overweight child achieve a normal weight; mom will have a healthier pregnancy; siblings will get better grades or excel in sports. It's good for everyone: one family, one approach. Pick your favorite cliché. You get the picture.

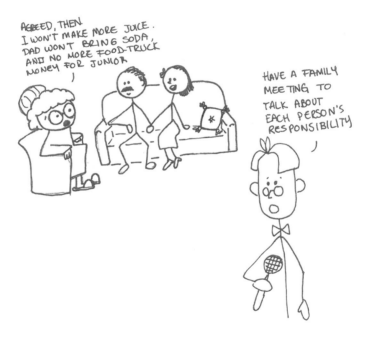

Communication

Communication is much more than the words we speak. Think about what else you might be communicating to your child through your actions, inactions, or body language. Communication has to be clear and consistent. Once you decide what the rules are, stick to them. One parent cannot waltz in with junk food. If Dad makes a sour face every time asparagus is put on the table, the child will learn that asparagus tastes bad before he or she has even tried it—though this doesn't mean that you have to be overly rigid. There's nothing wrong with one of the rules being "let's not be fanatics about this," but the clearer you are about things, the better it will be for everyone. Perhaps the clearest message of all is that *no* should always and consistently mean no, and not, "Please take *no* as an invitation to start a long process of negotiation where you do your best to manipulate me, and I eventually cave in like I always do."

In other words, *no mixed messages.*

Communication is an art and the basis of every successful, harmonious relationship. Learning how to express your desires, expectations, opinions, and demands in a nonthreatening, nonjudgmental fashion is crucial. There's an amazing book on the subject, *Nonviolent Communication* by Marshall Rosenberg. It's a great read, and we highly recommend picking up a copy. The book offers simple, practical tools for expressing yourself in a way that allows other people to hear and understand you. Equally important, it gives you tools to better understand your child's method of communication and what it is he or she is really asking for and needing from you.

Whether you get a copy of the book or not, understand that communication doesn't always come naturally to everyone. Knowing how to hear and be heard is a skill, and once you become conscious of it and tune in to your patterns and methods of expressing yourself, as well as your child's patterns, you can start to hone these skills. Your children will be grateful, because even if they're not aware of it, they truly want a deeper, more meaningful connection with you. They just don't know how to go about getting it. Your improved communication skills can help give them the oppor-

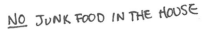
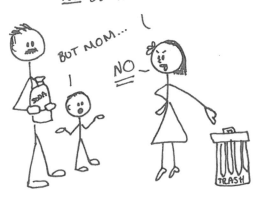

tunity to have that connection. The result: less stress, greater feelings of love and safety, more energy, more inspiration, a renewed desire to please you, and an increased desire to take care of themselves.

In Fit Club, we are committed to creating a safe environment where all children feel comfortable to exercise, so we have ground rules, like "no name-calling" and "always be encouraging to one another." Yet, not every child comes to us able to follow these rules. Many have been bullied themselves and will yell at their teammates, using derogatory statements about their weight. Our facilitators will pull them aside and redirect them, and soon they are kind, encouraging, and acting like good sports. They learn by watching how our staff treats the group, as well as how they keep kids in check when they are not acting appropriately. This also needs to happen in families. Siblings and parents should not be permitted to name call or bully. Words can cause deep and painful wounds. They should be used to lift each other up, not pull each other down.

Consistency

Another way of ensuring consistency is not to shift the goalposts. If you commit to something like eliminating junk food from the house, then don't suddenly decide that it's magically become okay because the supermarket is having a sale on candy this week. And if you promise to do something, like going for a walk after dinner, do it, unless there's a sudden thunderstorm. Consistency also applies to how various family members get treated, as well as other children.

You cannot afford double standards. Take the junk food example again: either every child can have junk food, or none of them can. How this works out depends on the specific circumstances of each family. A thin fifteen-year-old might resent having to deny himself potato chips for the sake of his twelve-year-old sister, but remember that it's not just for his sister's health; it's for his own health too. We've found many cases in which an underweight child is as unhealthy as an overweight child, and an improvement in the quality of food in the household is going to have benefits for all the family members across the board, which brings us to . . .

The Food in the House

When kids are younger, they have no purchasing power, so you have much more control over the foods that are available to them. When they're older, it's more challenging. But at the very least, you can stock the refrigerator, freezer, and pantry with a healthy range of foods that every member of the family has equal access to. We'll review the specifics again of what kinds of food to stock in your home in the next chapter, but for now, it's important to realize that once you decide what those food options are, you should make them as available as your means will allow. This will minimize complaints, like "Jonny ate all my almonds!" We encourage three meals and two to three snacks a day, because this helps many people regulate their blood sugar far more effectively than only eating three meals a day.

Offering food frequently also gets rid of any scarcity mentality about food that might arise. Remember that making food available is often one way to help kids feel more food secure and ensure they are never in starvation mode.

Getting Mealtimes Right

We've mentioned this before, but it's worth emphasizing again that mealtimes are a tremendous opportunity for healing. Along with having a constant supply of healthy food options available, formal mealtimes are still an important part of most people's lives, and they provide an everyday opportunity to share our lives with our families. We'd even go as far as to say that the family that eats together, thrives together. Families that don't share mealtimes tend to resemble households made up of roommates rather than families. The sharing of meals really is a bonding experience. Mealtimes are the most important opportunity to reinforce the general principles that will help your overweight child.

There should be only one set of rules for the whole family. People within the family should not be singled out or given a specific meal plan, unless food allergies are in the mix. In fact, if food allergies are severe enough, those foods might need to be out of the house altogether. But practically speaking, don't allow one child to have cake because he ate this or that, regardless of his or her weight. Either everyone can have the cake—as much as he or she wants—or nobody can have cake. You won't be able to escape sibling rivalry altogether. It's just human nature for kids to compete for the attention and love of their parents. One thing you can do is to treat everyone equally, regardless of size.

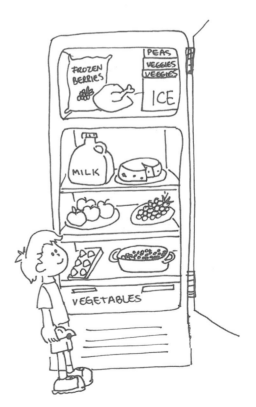

And don't rush things. At mealtimes your kids can get nourished at every level. When possible, create enough time for people to enjoy the food and each other's company. Sure, sometimes people are in a hurry. Sometimes meals compete with last-minute work deadlines, overscheduling, and other interruptions. Sometimes mealtimes can resemble World War III, but it doesn't have to be that way.

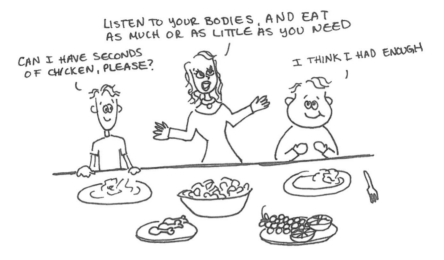

If mealtimes are not as great as they could be, a little bit of diagnosis might be in order. Maybe you need to find out, honestly, what mealtime means to you and your children. When your kids close their eyes and imagine dinnertime with the family, what do you think they see? What do they tell you that they see? What do you see? Is there a television on? Is there soda pop on the table? Chips? Are there fruits and vegetables around? Is there water? Are there brand names of packaged foods on the table? Does it look like a homemade picnic or more like a takeout dinner? Are people happy and laughing, or are they all staring at a television, barely engaging with their food or each other?

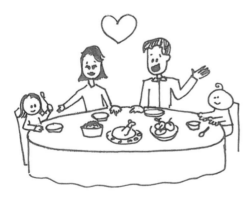

Which parts of these pictures do you like? What would you like to change? Don't be surprised if you all have different images about dinnertime and what it means. The point of these questions is to find out the difference between what you think you're creating with your kids and what you're actually creating. It also provides you with an opportunity to start creating something new—a time when you're all together, sharing and enjoying the food and each other's company.

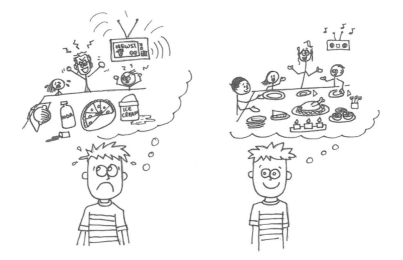

It's not all about food. Everything that you create in the home should be about creating a general feeling of safety and well-being. The home is supposed to be a refuge and place of safety. It's also supposed to be a place where kids can rely on you to be there for them. Unfortunately, in the world of single-parent families and demanding careers, children often come home to an empty house. We can't *always* devote the time we should to our kids; we can't always be there for them. Stuff happens. That's just life.

It's important to realize that the quality of the time you do spend with them is something you can control. So, if you are short on time, at the very least, take the time to make the moments with your child count.

Once again, it might be a good idea to compare the different mental pictures each member has of the family. When your kids close their eyes and imagine a fun time with Mom or Dad (or both), what are you all doing? Is there junk food or healthy food? Are you creating things or just consuming things? Are you physically active or passive? What do you imagine they see? What do you see? What's wrong with these pictures, if anything? What's right? What would you fix? In other words, what are your kids' ideas of family fun?

When you create a warm, nurturing family environment, you create a place where your kids will feel safe enough to get healthy.

The Right Type of Neglect

One of the best ways to help kids overcome a weight problem is to get them focused on something else besides their bodies. This is a case in which, in spite of all of our talk about support, a certain amount of "neglect" can actually work. "Neglecting" attention to a weight problem is more effective than obsessing over it. You're taking care of a problem, but we suggest that you do not encourage your child to be overly focused on it.

We recommend de-emphasizing the problem. So throw away scales, tape measures, and measuring cups and stop counting calories, fat, carbs, and so on. In fact, no counting at all. Just keep the focus on health, fun, common interests, connecting, bonding, and nourishing.

De-emphasizing their weight problem will help build a child's self-esteem. If there's one thing that overweight kids tend to suffer from, it's feelings of poor self-esteem.[2] Feelings of self-esteem and self-worth go hand in hand with self-care and healthy choices, even at a young age. People with low self-esteem often feel that they don't matter, so why look after themselves? After all, why bother to look after something of no value? The more someone values themselves, the more the person will take care of themselves.

Self-Esteem

Building up your child's self-esteem is a very important part of actively nurturing your child's spirit. One way to build up a child is to believe in him or her. Catch your child being good, smart, or funny, and point it out. Point out and praise them for things that are non-food related. Say things like, "I like the color schemes in that painting you made. You're a really talented painter," or "I love the way you helped your sister with her homework. You were patient and you explained things clearly to her. You were a great teacher."

Kids, like adults, build self-esteem through taking on a challenge and experiencing success. It's as simple as that—in principle at least. Allow your children to build self-esteem in whatever areas they are interested in, whether it's sports, school, or hobbies. It doesn't matter what the interest is, as long as it's healthy, challenging, creative, measurable, and above all else, acknowledged.

If kids can see that after a bit of practice, they can kick a ball farther than they could before, get a tune right on a musical instrument, or solve a puzzle faster, they will experience significant triumphs. The wins don't have to be *big*. They just have to be there and be acknowledged.

And most importantly, at least in the beginning, you should ensure that your kids are measuring their successes against their own personal bests. They need to feel that they're winning against themselves and that they have power over their own lives.

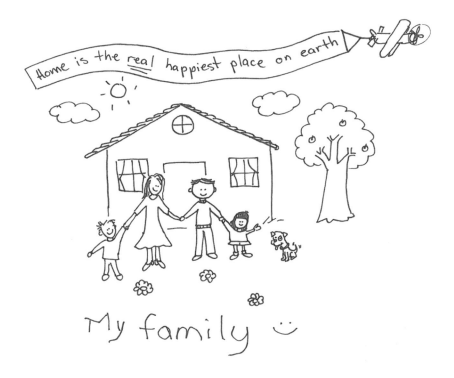

The hours you give your kids don't need to be a big production. Kids want the presence of their parents more than bells and whistles. Simply sharing time is more important than going to Disneyland. No matter what Disneyland might tell you, with a little work, home can be the happiest place on Earth for your child.

13

Bringing It All Together

At this point, you are armed with lots of new information that you're trying to process, and you've also got a few paradigm shifts to get used to. To make things easier and to help you get started, let's review some of the most important points we've discussed in the book so far. You can use this chapter as your quick go-to guide when you want to make sure you're doing things right.

First, clear out all the sugary drinks and the processed food from your home. Get rid of refined vegetable oils. Processed grains, like white rice, macaroni, and white flour, can be used for crafts if you don't want to throw them out or give them away. Use food coloring and string macaroni to make a fun necklace or bracelet. Glue rice on paper to give texture to artwork, or use white flour to make papier mâché or figurines. Add water to cornstarch to make glue.

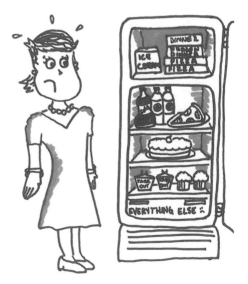

Now, find healthy foods to replace the processed food and restock your house. (Eat before you go shopping. You don't want to go shopping with a growling stomach because you'll crave junk food to increase your blood sugar.) You should fill your house with real foods—foods that existed in the caveman days, like fresh fruits, vegetables, green leafy salads, raw nuts and seeds, grass-fed meat, free-range chicken, wild-caught fish, and eggs.

Here's a good example of a well-balanced shopping list:

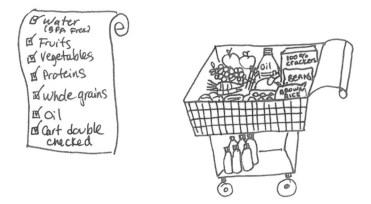

- **Fruits and vegetables:** Look for fresh fruits and vegetables that are in season. Try to get the most natural forms, and go organic when possible. Locally grown, spray-free fruits and vegetables are also good. Visit your local farmer's market, health food store, and co-op. Look particularly for produce to pack in lunch boxes and snacks on the go. Lunch-box fruits and vegetables have to be hearty to endure the wear and tear of being on the go. Examples include: carrots, broccoli, cucumbers, jicama, cherry tomatoes, oranges, apples, and bananas. If you can find sturdy, manageable containers, then you can try berries, cut melon, and salads.
- **Proteins:** Nuts (only if the child is old enough to chew them and not choke), nut butters, seeds, beans (including hummus), free-range eggs, grass-fed beef, free-range chicken, and wild-caught fish.
- **Healthy fats and oils:** Remember, some oils are ideal for cooking, and some oils should only be served cold. Good cooking oils include: ghee (or clarified butter), cold-pressed coconut oil, cold-pressed seed oil, and butter (preferably organic). Oils that are super healthy, but should only be served cold, include: flaxseed oil, chiaseed oil, and hempseed oil. These are great because they are high in omega-3 fatty acids, essential for reducing inflammation and turning off the FAT switch. You can use them as salad dressings or add them to smoothies. These oils should be cold-

pressed and kept refrigerated. We also recommend buying chia seeds to add to salads and smoothies.

Extra-virgin, cold-pressed olive oil is a great oil too, to serve cold or drizzle on vegetables. Avocados and avocado oil are great sources of healthy fats. And coconuts and coconut milk are also good sources of healthy fats.

- **Grains:** Grains and their benefits to human nutrition are very controversial, so at the very least, ensure that the grains you eat are unprocessed, 100 percent whole grains without added sugar. If you are sensitive to gluten or trying to eliminate gluten, good grain alternatives include: quinoa, spelt, buckwheat, kamut, and almond meal. You can use chia bran, flax meal, hemp meal, and coconut flour for baking things like muffins, breads, pancakes, crepes, and pizza dough. You can use *nori* sheets to make wraps. Nori is the seaweed used to make sushi rolls. It's loaded with healthy trace minerals and calcium.

- **Drinks:** Drink water (spring water or filtered water) at home. Put water in containers to take with you if you're going out, as long as the containers aren't contaminated with BPA. Herbal teas are also good. Chamomile or peppermint teas are mild and child-friendly.

- **Salt:** Replace table salt with sea salt, Himalayan salt crystals, volcanic salt, or Celtic salt. While salt has always gotten a bad rap, the truth is we need trace minerals in our diet, and healthy salt, in moderation, is a great way to get those trace minerals.

- **Fermented foods:** These are foods that are high in friendly bacteria, and as we've said many times, intestinal health is an important key to physical health. Recommended fermented foods include: unsweetened yogurts and kefirs made out of coconut milk, nut milk, or dairy; sauerkraut and kimchi; tempeh; miso; tamari; brewer's yeast; pickles; and so on. You can add these foods to wraps and salads.

Visit TheGabrielMethod.com/FitKids and DrRibasHealthClub.org /FitKids for lots of recipes on yummy ways to prepare all these real, "caveman" foods!

In a perfect world, you would fill your house with natural, seasonal, caveman-type foods and serve them at all meals and snacks. These foods should be unprocessed, unsweetened, and not fried. If you keep it seasonal, you'll offer a natural variety of foods, keep costs down, and have foods at their most tasty.

M
E
A
L
S

S
N
A
C
K
S

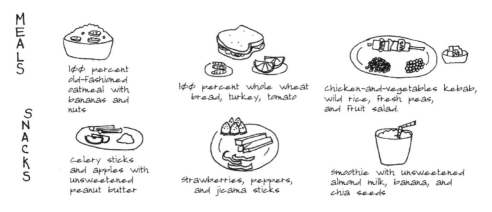

100 percent old-fashioned oatmeal with bananas and nuts

100 percent whole wheat bread, turkey, tomato

chicken-and-vegetables kebab, wild rice, fresh peas, and fruit salad.

Celery sticks and apples with unsweetened peanut butter

Strawberries, peppers, and jicama sticks

Smoothie with unsweetened almond milk, banana, and chia seeds

Use the seasons to not only inspire shopping lists and meal planning, but also to inspire family activities and exercise.

Meal Planning

You should serve three meals and two to three snacks a day to children over one year of age. Don't forget, it is your job to offer a variety of food. Simply eating a bowl of fruit for breakfast, regardless of how many types of fruit are in it, is not recommended. You need to add a protein, like nuts, a hard-boiled egg, a green shake, or plain yogurt. Add chia seeds to anything, like yogurts, salads, or shakes to provide omega-3 fatty acids. You are responsible for what is being served and when, so feed often. Children have small tummies, so we recommend offering food every two to three hours. Don't forget that regardless of what you serve, the child is responsible for deciding if, and how much, she will eat. Even after offering different food groups, she still may only eat the fruit. As long as you serve a variety of foods, you get a gold star. Sit down with your children and offer yourself a variety too. That cup of coffee is not going to cut it. Start planning your meals to include a fruit and a vegetable. Some examples include: egg, spinach, sliced peaches or a green shake, blueberries, and raw oatmeal (sweeten with unsweetened applesauce and sprinkle with cinnamon and chia seeds).

Snacks should include two to three food groups, ideally a fruit, a vegetable, and one additional group. One snack should be offered between breakfast and lunch and another should be offered after school, between lunch and dinner. If the child is still hungry after dinner, an additional snack or leftovers from dinner should be offered. A healthy snack could be: peanut butter with apples and celery; strawberries, carrots, and string cheese; or strips of red pepper with guacamole or hummus dip and a side of berries and cashews.

Water should be offered first thing in the morning, during each meal, each snack, and in between all snacks and meals.

Exercise Suggestions

Have a pillow fight in the morning or at night, have children participate in after-school sports, take after-dinner walks, or have dance competitions after a meal.

Bowtie & the Active Family

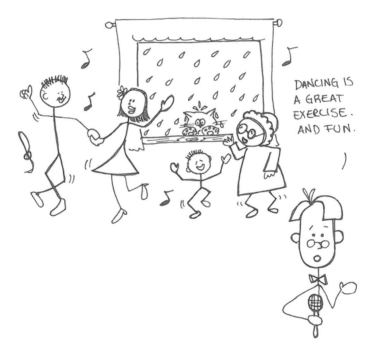

Bedtime

Savor this time with your children. This is one of the most important times of all. Always remember to read to your children or do an evening visualization with them.

If visualization becomes a daily, routine habit, it will help everything else fall into place. Once the mind changes, everything else follows.

There are several methods of visualization:

- Read a story to your child.
- Have your child listen to a pre-recorded story.
- Make up your own story, and tell it live or pre-record it for later.
- If your child is older, or if he or she just happens to have a talent for visualization, they can tell themselves a story they know or make one up as they go along.

How to Start

In the beginning, it can be quite daunting to try to put it all together. So start by making some small changes, like adding more real foods, developing a nighttime stress reduction and visualization ritual with your child, finding some playtime after school, and using mealtimes as a time to connect as a family. With these small steps, your child will be better nourished, have less stress, crave fewer sweets, and burn fat more efficiently.

We are both deeply committed to helping solve the very tragic yet preventable epidemic known as obesity. We need to get the word out and change the world's inaccurate and detrimental view toward weight, diets, and feeding children.

The beauty of our philosophy is that it promotes stronger relationships, playtime, and natural foods and reverts back to basic concepts we have all gotten away from in this modern world we live in. We are excited to send you off to enjoy family meals and for your whole family to become healthier.

By starting in this way, you'll be joining hundreds of thousands of people, in sixteen languages and sixty countries, who have discovered that weight loss and sustainable fitness is not about dieting and restriction, but instead, it's about health—real mind-body health.

As your child begins losing weight, their confidence will surge, and they'll start taking their health into their own hands. They'll be the ones asking for the salads and nutritious foods and being physically active on their own. Once they see the positive changes in their bodies and realize that they have the power to be fit in a sustainable way, you'll see a tremendous change, and the positive momentum will take over in their lives. Gone will be the child who sneaks candy when no one's looking, and in their place will be a child who is extremely motivated to succeed. When that happens, you've done your job, because you've given your child all the tools they need to be fit, healthy kids who grow up to become fit, healthy, happy, and successful adults.

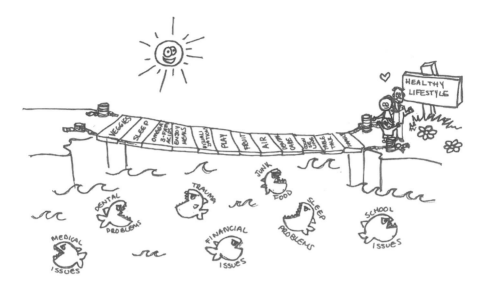

Connect with us at the web links www.TheGabrielMethod.com/FitKids and www.DrRibasHealthClub.org/FitKids, where you'll find recipes, snack ideas, visualization ideas, help for making mealtime fun, current news and tips, and anything and everything we can do to help you and your child reach your health and fitness goals.

Acknowledgments

Jon

This was a labor of love for so many of us. And the list of people that helped bring this work into fruition is too numerous to mention here. However, there are some people who I need to especially acknowledge.

First and for most, I'd like to thank Patricia and her amazing team for their tireless work and dedication, particularly Melinda Verissimo for her writing, editing, and research and Gabriela Menendez for her beautiful illustrations. Xavier Waterkeyn for his writing and editing brilliance. Our Barcelona team, including Lucas Rockwood, Sherri Kronfeld, Geraldine Navarrette, and Janine Oliver, as well as Anna, Hannah, and Sean for all of their vision in bringing this all together. Kelly Tomkies for her editing work. Oona Mansour for her creative recipes and innovative parenting ideas and for her hard work and dedication on the initial manuscript. Sharon Humphreys for her editing suggestions. And the team at Beyond Words for making it happen.

I'd also like to thank Rafi Nasser, Robert Peng, Daphne Goldberg, Jonathan Dichter, Khaliah and Jacob Ali, Spencer Wertheimer, James Colquhoun, Laurentine Ten Bosch, Prince Hugo Gabriel Colquhoun, Leonard, Ethel, Jennifer, Joe and Michelle Abrams, and Helen Duhigg. The brilliant and innovative doctors in the world that have helped us understand the real issues relating to childhood obesity, such as Dr. Mark Hyman, Dr. Joseph Mercola, Dr. Christian Northrup, Dr. Ronald Rosedale, Dr. Howard Leibowitz, and Donna Gates, to name a few.

Our Gabriel Method coaches: Brian Killian, Nealon Hightower, Christine Kennedy, Tracy Whitton, Melinda Jacobs, Heather Fleming, Jennifer Welch, Paula Robbins, Paul North, Smita Patel, Marjolijn Loderichs, Désirée Manders, and the rest of the Dutch coaching team. My own personal staff: Denaleigh Beard, Jenny Blackburn, Aeron McFarlane, Shannon Hawkes, and Mike Travers. I am so grateful for your dedication and support. Lastly, I'd like to thank the thousands of students we have around the world, who have helped us formulate and perfect the Gabriel Method principles—you continue to inspire me daily.

Dr. Patricia

I would like to thank my parents, who have always believed in me, which really did make a difference. My dad, who works harder than anyone I know and kept me putting one foot in front of the other, and my mom, who taught me to always dream big and the sky is the limit.

Desiree, my sister, my photographer, artist, and help—with Ashley and life in general. Aaron, her husband, my favorite Ultimate Boarder and someone who is always there for me.

My other sister, Valerie, the other Auntie Mommy, who has been a great source of inspiration and resourcefulness as we raise our girls together. You have the best style and the best ideas for cooking and gardening that I know. AJ, my brother-in-law, who has been so supportive. And my beautiful and diverse nieces, Ava and Lily.

Lucas, for bringing Jon and I together.

Jon, for being true to your word in every way and becoming a dear friend quickly. I love what you do, how you do it, and who you are while you do it. You are a pleasure to work with and know.

Xavier, the first pompous Australian I ever met, and now my favorite Australian. You are brilliant and I adore you.

Henry and Lindsay from Beyond Words, who have been so easy to work with.

My dream team, who work with their hearts on their sleeves every day in the trenches with me, driven by the passion to help others, compelled to make a difference in the families we care for, and creatively weaving pathways to bridge families from where they are to where they need to be. I am in awe of the way you are there for our patients, families, and each other and am so grateful for the personal support you give me as a friend. Every day I feel so blessed to work with you and amazed that you let me lead you. I get these ideas and you elaborate on them, make them better and then carry them to fruition. You are all amazing and are the wind beneath my wings

Gaby, who has been there from the start, my co-pilot, my Dr. Watson. You make things happen. You care for my patients, their families, and staff like family. There is nothing you can't do, from medicine to management to art. Yes, art, from murals in my clinic to illustrations for this book. There is no one as capable of so much as you. You have been such a blessed friend and partner in serving our community.

Melinda, I could not have written this book without you. You are a fantastic writer, and you always amaze me. You are so clever and hardworking and a joy to know. I will always be indebted to you for helping me write this book, as well as all the research you put into it. You go above and beyond expectations in everything you do, and you are never overwhelmed. You have kept me sane when there was so much to do.

Brandon, from Fast Twitch to the clinic, I have never heard you say anything bad about anyone. I have never seen you give less than 100 percent. Thank you for your expertise in helping with the exercise portion of this book.

Jennifer Nelson, the RD who taught me everything I know about nutrition. You spoon-fed me all of those pearls of knowledge in the most unassuming way. You have been a blessing to know and work with, and I stand on your shoulders every day.

Rosario, my go-to girl for everything and anything. What a treasure to have such a resource in my life and on my team.

Vida you have been such an amazing addition to the team. You have been an awesome partner for me and a wonderful sounding board.

Karla you are so good to our patients. You are smart and compassionate. You are a great chef, fitness trainer, and medical assistant, and are always a source of creative ideas to help our patients and for the book.

Katy, our new RD, but immediately in the thick of things as a source of knowledge and compassion to our team and patients and helping with this book.

The rest of the team who supported me while we wrote this book: Stacy, Diana, Jennifer C., Crystal, Tommy, Ashley, Jason, Caitlin, Christie, and Kara Pitkin.

Joanne Christopherson, PhD, our awesome statistician who finds ways to help her UCI students learn while she helps us evaluate our care.

The Fast Twitch crew, who inspire and support me and make working out so enjoyable. We are more than friends. Dr. Tommy Knox, our fearless leader, Tom Tumbleson (the most generous man I know), Tyler, Adam, AJ, Tom Knapp, and Bob my favorite triathlete. Kerri and Casey Jennings, our amazing and genuine celebrity couple.

My dear friends who are always there for me through thick and thin, no matter what state they are living in or what is going on in their own lives: Trish Halvorsan, Julie O'Sullivan, Pam Porzio, and Christa Preston.

Peter, for supporting me through this process and others.

My incredible mentor: Dr. Gwyn Parry, the Marcus Welby of Corona del Mar who has guided my career from the beginning. You have helped me pursue my passions in community medicine and have always been there with resources for my patients. You have been there for me in all facets of my life, and I will always be grateful.

The Children and Families Commission of Orange County, who have believed in my program and supported my team solidly. Some specific people who have gone above and beyond to help me go from being inspired to help my patients to serving my community: Illia Rolon, Mike Ruane, Kim Goll, Sally Snyder, and Lisa Burke.

My colleagues and dear friends in community medicine: Albert, Miles, Eva, Pete, Debbie, Cyndie, and Becky.

My special teachers: Ted Bandruck, who taught us about life and community while we swam; Doug Volding, that coach who cared on and off the field and pool; Mr. Gillis, my high school English teacher who helped me write my medical school essay and died before I could tell him I got in and thank him; Mr. Dale Ghere, my high school biology teacher who first made me feel like a scientist; and my advisors at USC, who helped me long after graduation—Dr. Don Batstone and the late Dr. Harry Kurtz, FIGHT ON!

Those who helped me get into medical school at BUSM: Dr. Broitman and my amazing advocate, Dr. Daniel Bernstein. Miltos and Simon, my study partners. Dr. Heike Rolle-Daya, my greatest role model as a mother and pediatrician and how to balance it all in life and medicine.

The incredibly compassionate and brilliant doctors at CHOC where I did my residency: Dr. Minion, who first taught me the path to go beyond the normal walls of medicine, and has continued to support me. Dr. Michael Muhonen, who was such an amazing neurosurgeon and human being that I wanted to learn from him. Dr. Dahr, my advisor, and all of the PSF, ER, and Out Patient doctors who trained me in pediatrics and role modeled compassion. Dr. Anita Sinha and Dr. Shirin Noorani, who both taught me community medicine. My colleagues, especially: Albert Chang, my scarecrow who started with me at BU, trained with me at CHOC, worked with me at HBCC, shot twenty-six episodes of *Doctor Doctor* with me, and has always been there for me in every way.

Dr. Jack Shohet, my compassionate ENT who was so good to me when I lost my hearing and battled vertigo. He reminded me how a doctor should be when someone is vulnerable, scared, feeling lousy, and powerless. Teresa England, PT, who also helped me recover.

My collaborators and supporters: Allergan Foundation; CalOptima, Dr. Carter, Linda Lee, and Sandra Rose; Chase the Stars Foundation and Kerri Walsh Jennings, who has been a dear friend and great supporter of our program; Child Guidance Center, Lori Pack and Dr. Marta Shinn; Children and Families Commission of Orange County; Donnie Crevier; Harvard Institute of Coaching; Healthy Smiles; Hoag Memorial Hospital; HOPE Clinic and NMUSD RNs, Merry, Audrey, Laura, and Annette; Kaiser Permanente, Cheryl Vargo, Mary, and Dick Allen; Mission Hospital, Judi Kennard; Nestle Waters (Pat O'Sullivan); OC Cares (Dr Ahn), Orange County Community Foundation (Shelley Hoss, Todd Hanson), and OneOC (Dan and Valerie); Orangewood Children's Home, Jaimie Munoz and Dr. Liz Ligason; Pretend City, Sandra Bolton; San Juan Pediatrics, Dr. Fahim; Sisters of St. Joseph Healthcare Foundation, Sister Regina Fox; St. Joseph Health System Foundation, Gabriela Robles; Tanaka Farms; Toys for Tots; Weingart Foundation; Wells Fargo Foundation; Whole Foods Newport Beach, Cindy O'Shea; and the YMCA.

My favorite preschool directors, Lynette Anderson and Courtenay Conzelman. My daughter's and my favorite kindergarten teacher, Mrs. Archibald, who lets me bring new programs to her class at Harbor View Elementary School.

My dear friends through Illumination Foundation and onward: the Two Pauls, Yvette Cabrera, Scott Smith, and Jack Toan.

My friends at Nordstrom's in Fashion Island: Melissa Morris, Brittney Bartholomew, and Beth Willis, as well as my dear Trevor at Spa Gregorie's, who all worked to make me look presentable for this book.

My awesome Fit Scout Troop. Every meeting you remind me how wonderful, smart, and sweet children are and how you will all make this world a better place in the next generation: Ashley (my inspiration and co-captain), Aaliyah, Aven, Brooke, Ella, Isabelle, Jacqui, Jayna, Kelsey, Makenna, Olivia, Samantha B, Samantha T, Shea, and Sophia. As well as the adults helping us: Stacy (our leader), Kara, Jill, Christa, and CC.

The Angels, who I carry in my heart every day. I am a better person to have known you and your families. You are remembered and adored: Kim Kikuchi, Skyler Aarvig, and Jonathan Pollitt.

My dear patients and their fabulous families: I won't betray your confidence by naming you, but I am so grateful to you for trusting me and my team and telling your stories and struggles and stresses, and allowing me to care for you. I have learned so much from you all and feel blessed to be your doctor.

Appendix I:
Visualizations

There Are So Many Kisses:
For Younger Children

Butterflies kiss lash to lash
Kissing fish pair up and dash

Eskimos kiss to warm a nose
Kissing bugs peck when you doze

Angel kisses mark baby's face
Grooms kiss brides in a wedding embrace

Kissing booths are at the fair
Kissing bandits are quick, beware

You can hope for a prince and kiss a frog
Or get a wet face from a kissing dog

Hugs and kisses (XOXO) end a letter
But a sweet dreams kiss is even better . . .
Good night

Good Night
(Dreaming Tree Revisited):
For Early School-Aged Children

Under a great welcoming moon . . . stands a dreaming tree, outside your room

Its leaves packed with rainbows, which never fade . . . A talking clock, a hero made

A baby's feet touching—giggles and bubbles and curls . . . as you ride huge butterflies flying in swirls

Majestic horses and dueling swords, adventurers traveling through different worlds

Take a rest at its feet, pull a blanket, for tea . . . and sip and enjoy with fresh berries and glee

Flowers floating all around and natural springs flowing up from the ground

A yummy vegetable sits all shiny and bright . . . and lends nourishment you need for the night

Climb, climb high, each branch is a journey, each leaf a favorite memory formed in a hurry

The night air is fresh, flapping through your pajamas, and wholesome and rare as you skate with four llamas

Then costumes will drape you to keep you warm, which sparkle brightly, woven with all that adorn

You can't help but smile, in this luscious tree, light wings from your shoulders, you feel so free

Higher and higher and higher you go, dancing, and flying and whirling you flow

Sing like a bird, an angel, whatever tune you form . . . the dreaming tree will be there and bring you right home

The dreaming tree is peaceful and calm, storing your wishes, your shovels . . . your pond

It soothes your heart, wipes your tears . . . it fills your hope with all that cheers

Possibilities are endless in that dreaming tree outside, smiling at the moon, your imagination will glide

You are safe; you are happy; you are strong and quick, as the hands of the clock gently tick . . . Savor your dreams, your hope, your might and reach, reach, reach for the stars tonight . . .

Good night

The Green Street Warriors:
For School-Aged Boys

So we're going to go on a little journey. Now, I'd like you to imagine that you walk outside, and there's a group of guys waiting to see you, and they're very powerful, tall, strong, and determined—really cool looking guys. And one of them walks up to you and says, "We're the Green Street Warriors, and we're going to take you for a ride." And when you look at him, you can see that he's powerful, but at the same time, he's going to take care of you; all these guys are. And you get on their motorcycles, and you go for a ride. Some of them are riding in front of you, some of them are riding beside you, and there's a few riding behind you. And you're in the middle, on the back of a motorcycle, and you're riding down the street. People are watching you, and they see how powerful these guys are. Everyone is impressed with these guys, and they're there to take care of you and to take you on a journey.

They go faster and faster, and then all of a sudden they go so fast that they start going into the air. You soar into the sky, into the night sky, and you see the city and towns below you, and you feel the wind in your hair. And you're holding on, and it just feels amazing. You soar up past the sky, into space, and you just keep flying on these motorcycles to another place, to another land.

You can see in the distance a planet, a beautiful, blue planet, very similar to Earth, and you can see that that's where you're heading. And the man who's on the motorcycle with you says, "We're going to take you to meet our leader." You go flying into the sky, and you go into the atmosphere, and you land on this planet, on a tropical island on the sand. And you get off the bikes, and you go for a walk with these guys, and they're circling all around you to protect you and guide you. You can see how strong they are, how determined they are, but at the same time, they've got your back. They're not going to let anything happen to you.

They take you through the jungle, to this beautiful palace made out of marble, gold, stone, diamonds, and silver. And you start walking up the marble stairs to the top of this palace, and as you take each step, you know that something powerful is about to happen. You know something very real is about to happen. And you walk farther and farther and farther up the stairs, until you reach this beautiful, big opening, and there's a very tall, muscular, powerful man waiting to see you, a warrior with long hair and a necklace made of bones.

You walk up to him and he must be seven feet tall, or over two meters high. He's so tall, like a world-class basketball player, and he's muscular, lean, powerful, and determined. And you can see his face, his chiseled face and his eyes; he's got eyes of steel and glass. He looks at you and says, "I'm the leader of the Green Street Warriors, and I am the most powerful person on this planet. My power is infinite, and there's nothing I can't do." And he says, "I'm going to give you my power, because I've got so much of it. I can give you all that I want, and so I'm going to give you everything you need and more," and he grins at you.

As he's radiating this power into your body, you can feel your body changing. Your body's getting lean and fit and powerful. You feel the power in your bones. You feel this power going into your legs, your arms, your wrists, your back, your ribs, your shoulders, and your head, power just being radiated into your body, and it feels so amazing. The confidence, his confidence, becomes your confidence, and you feel your body getting healthier and healthier and healthier. Everywhere that his power goes, in every part of your body, it heals your body, it re-energizes it, and you feel this incredible sense of confidence and security. And he says to you, "With this power that I'm giving you, with this energy that I'm giving you, you now have all the power in the world to do whatever you want. You have the power to be amazingly successful in sports and in school and in any dreams you have."

You can see yourself playing sports, loving them, and being a champion in any sport that you want, easily and effortlessly scoring the goal, winning the game, running the race. You can see your body getting fitter and healthier, and you can see the confidence that's now in you. And he says, "With this power, you can be as successful as you could ever possibly imagine at school," and you see yourself easily and effortlessly acing any exam, getting straight As, and rising to the top, and it's easy, and it's effortless.

He says to you, "With this power, you have the power to love healthy, vibrant foods that will continue to make your body more and more powerful." And you can see yourself during the day craving healthy, vibrant foods, real foods, the types of foods that nature intended you to eat, the types of foods that make you powerful beyond your wildest imagination.

As he continues to keep his hand on your forehead, radiating this energy into your body, he says to you, "With this power, you have all the energy you need to be successful in every area of your life. Hobbies, music, jobs, work, social life, anything, and you can see yourself being tremendously successful." "And with this energy," he says to you, "you now have the power to be effortlessly fit, healthy, and happy," and you see yourself getting fitter and fitter, and your most strong and healthy body. You see yourself effortlessly getting fitter and fitter, stronger, and more powerful, more confident, more secure, and more successful in every aspect of your life.

And he takes his hand off of your forehead, he puts his hands on your shoulders, and he just looks at you, and you feel a combination of love, acceptance, security, power, wisdom, and knowledge, and he says, "I will always protect you. I will always be there for you. I will always be radiating my power, my energy, into you, to give you all the energy you need to be successful, healthy, strong, and happy. I will always be there for you, and you will be successful beyond your wildest imagination."

As he has his hands on your shoulders, you can see your body starting to transform into the body that you truly want to have. And you're strong, happy, healthy, secure, and ready to live a tremendously successful life in every possible way. And you just look at each other, and you nod, and then you turn and walk away, and the Green Street Warriors take you back to their bikes. Back on the shore, you go flying into the air effortlessly and enjoyably, back to planet Earth. And they let you off at your door, and you come back to bed, and you lay there and allow yourself to drift off to sleep, knowing that you now have all the energy you need, now and always, to feel safe, confident, secure, and powerful. You have all the energy you need and you'll be tremendously successful at school, in your social life, in sports, and in every area of your life. You will radiate health, happiness, security, success, and fitness beyond your wildest imaginations.

And now you allow yourself to drift off to sleep, knowing that tomorrow, you're going to have one of the most amazing days of your life, and you're going to get healthier, happier, fitter, more secure, more confident, and more successful, now and always, in every area of your life.

The Horse Clan of the Amazons: For School-Aged Girls

So we're going to go on a little journey. Now, I'd like you to imagine that you walk outside, and there's a group of women waiting to see you, and they're very powerful, tall, strong, determined—really cool looking women. And one of them walks up to you and says, "We're the Amazons, and we're going to take you for a ride." And when you look at her, you can see that she's powerful, but at the same time, she's going to take care of you; all these women are. You see that they're all riding these beautiful horses. Some of them are riding in front of you, some of them are riding beside you, and there's a few riding behind you.

And you're in the middle, on the back of a beautiful horse, and you're galloping down the street. People are watching you, and they see how powerful these women are, and everyone is in awe of these women, and they're there to take care of you and take you on a journey.

They go faster and faster, and then all of a sudden they go so fast that they start going into the air, and you soar into the sky, into the night sky, and you see the city and towns below you, and you feel the wind in your hair. And you're holding on, and it just feels amazing. You're all galloping up past the sky, into space, and you just keep flying on these horses to another place, to another land.

You can see in the distance a planet, a beautiful, blue planet, very similar to Earth, and you can see that that's where you're heading. The woman who's on the horse with you says, "We're going to take you to meet our leader." And you go flying into the sky, and you go into the atmosphere, and you land on this planet, in a tropical island on the sand. You get off the horses, and you go for a walk with these women, and they're circling all around you to protect you and guide you. And you can see how confident they are, how strong they are, how determined they are, but at the same time they've got your back. They're not going to let anything happen to you.

They take you through the jungle, to this beautiful palace made out of marble, gold, stone, diamonds, and silver. And you start walking up the marble stairs to the top of this palace, and as you take each step, you know that something powerful is about to happen. You know something very real is about to happen. And you walk farther and farther and farther up the stairs, until you reach this beautiful, big opening, and there's a very tall, lean, stronger, powerful woman waiting to see you, a warrior, with long hair and a necklace made of seashells.

You walk up to her, and she must be seven feet tall, or over two meters high. She's so tall, like a world-class basketball player, and she's lean, stronger, powerful, and determined. And you can see her face, her striking face and her eyes—eyes that look like they're carved from jewels. She looks at you, and she says, "I'm the leader of the Amazons, and I am the most powerful person on this planet. My power is infinite, and there's nothing I can't do." And she says, "I'm going to give you my power, because I've got so much of it. I can give you all that I want, and so I'm going to give you everything you need and more," and she smiles.

She puts her hand on your forehead, and you feel this radiation coming through her hand into your body. Power, the power of the universe going into your bones, and you feel this power going into your legs, your arms, your wrists, your back, your ribs, your shoulders, your head, and even your hair, power just being radiated into your body, and it feels so amazing and energizing.

As she's radiating this power into your body, you can feel your body changing. Your body's getting lean, stronger, fit, and powerful. You feel the power in your bones. The confidence, her confidence, becomes your confidence, and you feel your body getting healthier and healthier and healthier. Everywhere that her power goes, in every part of your body, it heals your body, it re-energizes it, and you feel this incredible sense of confidence and security. And she says to you, "With this power that I'm giving you, with this energy that I'm giving you, you now have all the power in the world to do whatever you want. You have the power to be amazingly successful in sports and in school and in any dreams you have."

You can see yourself playing sports, loving them, and being a champion in any sport that you want, easily and effortlessly scoring the goal, winning the game, running the race. And you can see your body getting fitter and healthier, and you can see the confidence that's coming out of you. She says, "With this power, you can be as successful as you could ever possibly imagine at school," and you see yourself easily and effortlessly acing any exam, getting straight As, and rising to the top, and it's easy and it's effortless.

As she continues to keep her hand on your forehead, radiating this energy into your body, she says to you, "With this power, you have all the energy you need to be successful in every area of your life. Hobbies, music, jobs, work, social life, anything, and you can see yourself being tremendously successful." "And with this energy," she says to you, "you now have the power to be effortlessly fit, healthy, and happy." You see yourself effortlessly getting fitter and fitter, stronger, more powerful, more confident, more secure, and more successful in every aspect of your life.

You look at her, you look her right in the eyes, and you say to her, "With this energy, I now have the power to be effortlessly fit, to be successful at school, at anything I try, and to be happy, healthy, confident, to love my life and to be successful in every area of my life."

And she takes her hand off of your forehead, she puts her hands on your shoulders, and she just looks at you, and you feel a combination of love, acceptance, security, power, wisdom, and knowledge, and she says, "I will always protect you. I will always be there for you. I will always be radiating my power, my energy, into you, to give you all the energy you need to be successful, healthy, fit, and happy. I will always be there for you, and you will be successful beyond your wildest imagination."

As she has her hands on your shoulders, you can see your body starting to change. And you find yourself standing there just like her, a true warrior in every sense of the word. And you're fit, happy, healthy, secure, and ready to live a tremendously successful life in every possible way. And you just look at each other and you nod, and then you turn and walk away, and the Amazon clan takes you back to their horses. Back on the shore, you go flying into the air effortlessly and enjoyably, back to planet Earth. They let you off at your door, and you come back to bed, and you lay there and allow yourself to drift off to sleep, knowing that you now have all the energy you need, now and always, to feel safe, confident, secure, and powerful. You have all the energy you need to be effortlessly fit and be tremendously successful at school, in your social life, in sports, and in every area of your life. You will radiate health, happiness, security, success, and strength beyond your wildest imaginations.

And now you allow yourself to drift off to sleep, knowing that tomorrow, you're going to have one of the most amazing days of your life, and you're going to get healthier, happier, fitter, more secure, more confident, and more successful, now and always, in every area of your life.

The White Light: For School-Aged Children

There is a white ball of light that glides over to you like a good friend. It is white, calm, peaceful, and warm and feels like a hug when it touches the tips of your toes. The white light travels through your feet as you breathe, making your muscles relax. This makes you feel calm and loved and safe.

The white light travels to your ankles and up to your knees, giving you the feeling of peace, calm, and tranquility in all that it touches, as it spreads gently up your body like a blanket. It travels to your hips and waist and then to your ribs and back. It makes you feel peaceful, calm, tired, and relaxed, and it stretches to your shoulders and down your arms to your elbows. You feel safe, peaceful, relaxed, and sleepy.

It spreads to your wrist and your hands and shoots through all ten of your fingers, as it soothes your body and makes you feel peaceful, calm, and ready to sleep. It goes up your neck and your jaw and relaxes everything it touches, then goes to your ears and cheeks, to the back of your head, making you feel calm, safe, sleepy, and peaceful. It travels over the back of your eyes, your nose, and forehead, spreading peaceful thoughts and making you feel relaxed.

Now, your whole body is filled with this white light, and you feel so peaceful, grateful, calm, and tired. You are falling asleep and ready to dream of flying with the stars and moon, seeing beautiful things on your adventure.

In the morning when you wake up, you will feel good and rested, and everything will be easy for you. You will easily get ready, finding just the right clothes to wear, and you will look and feel great. You will have breakfast and go to school, you will be early, and everything will come easily for you. You will learn so much at school, everything will make sense, and you will be so friendly and kind and make friends easily. You will have so much fun at recess with the other children, playing and laughing, and the day will be so enjoyable. You will feel so good, safe, strong, friendly, and smart. Little things will come up, but they won't be a big deal. They will work themselves out like they always do . . . it will be a great day tomorrow.

Appendix II: Seasonal Food Suggestions and Activities

As we touched on in chapter 3, being creative with meals is a great way to get your children eating nutritious food. In chapter 8, we showed just how important it is to foster an active lifestyle to stay both physically and mentally fit. In the following pages, we've provided four seasonally inspired sections to keep the entire family fit and healthy—winter, spring, summer, and fall.

Safety in the Kitchen

Preparing food can be a wonderful experience for parents and children, but before we begin, the following is a quick rundown of certain safety measures that need to be in place and understood in the kitchen in order to prevent illness or injury to junior chefs and the recipients of their food:

1. Always wash your hands with soap and water before cooking and before switching to a different food.
2. Once hands are washed, avoid touching your hair or skin. If you do, rewash hands.
3. Wash all knives, spoons, cutting boards, bowls, and so on before use and before using with a different food.
4. Use separate cutting boards and utensils for raw meats (you can use a sharpie to identify).
5. Be sure to cook all foods thoroughly and keep them at the right temperature (hot foods hot, cold foods cold).

6. Keep all perishable items in the refrigerator until just before use (like milk, eggs, meats and so forth).

7. Refrigerate leftovers immediately (if left out too long, it is best to throw them away).

8. For children under four years of age, avoid the following choking hazards: most nuts, like peanuts and almonds; hunks of raw fruits and vegetables, like carrots or grapes (unless chopped completely); and any other foods, like gum and popcorn.

9. Knives: many foods can be prepared and chopped with plastic knives, which are less likely to cut little fingers, but be sure to watch children carefully when they are chopping.

10. Pan handles and the stove: teach children to assume burners are always on and not to touch stove top. Turn handles away as they may be bumped or fall.

11. Potholders: parents should handle hot food, but children need to know where potholders are and how to use them.

Spring

The following are tips on using the spring to inspire healthy activities and nutrition for children and families.

Activities for Preschoolers/Toddlers

- Leap frog or ring-around-a-rosy
- Egg hunt: instead of filling plastic eggs with candy, use coins or have a golden ticket redeemable for a book, movie ticket, or other prize, like a small toy.
- Go on a walk or hike. If it's raining, put on rain boots, bring an umbrella, and have a fun walk in the rain.
- Make walks more fun for children by observing and discussing nature, like looking out for squirrels, birds, rabbits, and other wildlife. See who can name the most flowers and or collect the most interesting rocks.

Activities for School-Aged/Teens

- Play an active game of golf, basketball, or tennis. Families can make friendly wagers, like whoever wins doesn't have to do the dishes that night. You don't only have to play the full game to be active either. For golf, you can play a short game of three or nine holes, or try miniature or twilight golf where games are shorter. And if you're stuck inside or don't have access to something like a golf course, you can putt the ball around the house or on grass or use that croquet set that may have been collecting dust in the garage. If a more active sport like basketball is more your family's taste, practice layups together, or see how many free throws you can make in a row. Play a game of HORSE or Around-the-World with a friend. Or for tennis, see how long you can rally the ball back and forth and try to beat that each round.

- Egg hunts and scavenger hunts are also effective with school-aged kids and even teens, but again, don't merely fill the eggs with junk food; find other small toys or prizes that your kids will like; create an engaging experience and provide nutritious food for the family.

Spring-Inspired Nutrition

- Apricots
- Artichokes
- Asparagus
- Broccoli
- Corn
- Green beans
- Honeydew
- Mangos
- Oranges
- Peas
- Radishes
- Strawberries

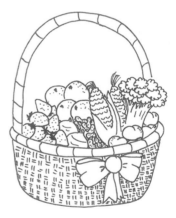

Tea parties: Great for holidays like Mother's Day, tea parties are made more fun with costumes, like hats and boas. Steep chamomile or mint tea in a tea pot and then have smaller cups for the children to drink from. Put a small bowl of crushed ice that the children can spoon into tea if it's too hot for them. There's no need to have sugar or honey on the table; the ice and fresh mint will be fine. Include fresh berries, cut melon, peanuts, or popcorn (for children over four years) to munch on.

Spring basket: Color hardboiled eggs with food dye. On a plate, place leaves of lettuce with a thin layer of shredded carrots on top. Once both layers are set, place your colorful egg over carrots. Afterwards, peel and slice the eggs and enjoy a healthy, protein-rich salad.

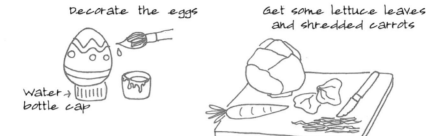

Decorate the eggs

Water → bottle cap

Get some lettuce leaves and shredded carrots

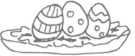

Place your eggs on top of a lettuce/carrots bed

*Remember to ask an adult for help whenever you are cutting, slicing, or peeling.

Summer

The following are tips on using the summer to inspire healthy activities and nutrition for children and families (Be sure to serve lots of water on hot days. You can also make tea and refrigerate it for a refreshingly cool, healthy drink):

Activities for Preschoolers/Toddlers
- Play hide-and-go seek.
- Play a game of "freeze dancing," playing music outside or in the house that children dance to until you stop the music, in which case they must stop dancing. This is a great game for this age group, and children love it!
- Run in the front yard with a sprinkler or a hose to cool off.

Activities for School-Aged/Teens
- Practice throwing a baseball around or have members of the family take turns at bat.
- Tag: play different variations of tag, like freeze tag, tunnel tag, and cartoon tag.
- Capture the flag.
- Go for a swim.

• Fill up water balloons and have a water balloon game, or play tag with squirt guns

Summer-Inspired Nutrition

• Apricots
• Beets
• Bell peppers
• Blackberries
• Blueberries
• Cantaloupe
• Cherries
• Corn
• Cucumbers
• Eggplant
• Figs
• Green beans
• Melon
• Nectarines
• Peaches
• Plums
• Radishes
• Raspberries
• Tomatoes
• Watermelon
• Zucchini

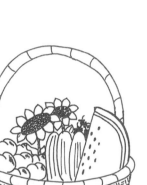

Fruits: Take advantage of all the fruit in season this time of year and make them more fun by using a melon baller to scoop out watermelon, cantaloupe, and honeydew. Presentation is everything, so even accessorize the plate with fun umbrella toothpicks. Children will eat it up!

Hot-day cool down: Frozen grapes, pineapple, cucumbers, almonds, and watermelon—all make cooling snacks that really hit the spot on a hot day. Or put a banana on a stick and freeze it. Then heat up peanut butter and roll the frozen banana in it, along with some cut up dates (optional), and freeze.

Backyard BBQs: Add onions, tomatoes, bell peppers, and pineapple to skewers for a grilled veggie option.

Ladybugs: Use a watermelon round to make the ladybug's body, small slices of a mozzarella for the eyes, and then add raisins attached to the ends of toothpicks as the antennae.

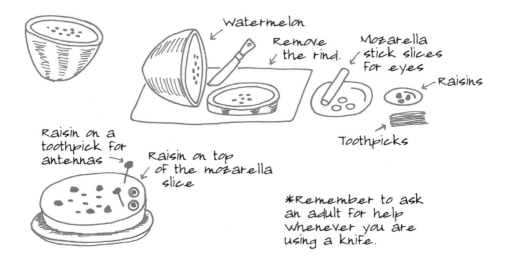

Fall

The following are tips on using the fall to inspire healthy activities and nutrition for children and families:

Activities for Preschoolers/Toddlers
- Go apple picking or visit a local pumpkin patch.
- Dance to Halloween-themed songs while dressed in costume.

Activities for School-Aged/Teenagers
- Throw the football around or play a game of soccer.
- Go for a hike.

Fall-Inspired Nutrition

- Acorn squash
- Apples
- Brussels sprouts
- Butternut squash
- Cauliflower
- Cranberries
- Grapes
- Mushrooms
- Pears
- Persimmons
- Pineapple
- Pomegranates
- Pumpkin
- Swiss chard
- Sweet potatoes
- Turnip

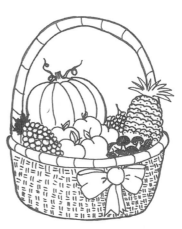

Halloween: Celebrate Halloween with black-and-orange snacks, like sunflower seeds, cuties (oranges), orange bell pepper slices, raisins, and sweet potatoes.

Make a Waldorf salad: Use a cup of cut apples, celery, pomegranate seeds, and walnuts. Squeeze lemon over the ingredients and serve cold with an autumn dinner.

Seasonal fare: Roast vegetables like cauliflower and butternut squash drizzled in grapeseed oil and sprinkled with salt and pepper. Cook at 350 degrees for 25 minutes, or until slightly crisp and brown.

Thanksgiving turkey: Make a fun turkey using a whole apple or pear for the body, thread raisins and/or orange wedges on toothpicks for the turkey's feathers, and raisins and a pimento olive for the face.

Apple   Toothpicks   Orange or   Raisins
                              tangerine
                              segments

Eyes (raisins on toothpicks)   Feathers (raisins, or orange
                                            segments on a toothpick)

(carrot, olive, or other
fruit on a toothpick)

*Remember to always ask an adult for help when
handling a kinfe, toothpicks, and other kitchenware.

Winter

The following are tips on using the winter to inspire healthy activities and
nutrition for children and families:

Activities for Preschoolers/Toddlers
- Make a snowman.
- Bundle up and go on a walk to see the neighborhood's holiday lights.

Activities for School-Aged/Teenagers
- Go ice skating, skiing, or sledding.
- Leave your wallet in the car and walk
  around the malls window shopping.

Winter-Inspired Nutrition
- Brussels sprouts
- Chestnuts
- Clementines
- Collard greens
- Dates
- Grapefruit
- Kale
- Kiwi

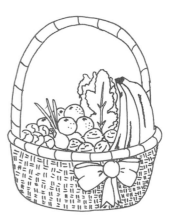

- Leeks
- Oranges
- Tangerines
- Turnips

Seasonal fare: Make roasted Brussels sprouts or chestnuts for a heart-warming snack.

Salt dough ornaments: One way to get rid of processed grains and enjoy the fun of the holidays is to make salt dough ornaments. This way, children will still be able to have all the fun of making cookies—measuring, cooking, and decorating—without putting the processed grains and sugars in their bodies. Once decorated, they can then hang them on a Christmas tree or give them out as gifts. Things you'll need:

- 1/2 cup salt
- 1 cup all-purpose flour
- 1/2 cup warm water
- Non-toxic acrylic paint
- Markers
- Flour sifter
- Cookie cutters
- Rolling pin
- Drinking straw
- Ribbons and glitter

1. Mix salt and flour together. Add water.
2. Knead dough until smooth. The dough should be very stiff. Add more flour if it's too sticky.
3. Roll dough out and cut ornaments with cookie cutters, or cut out your own figures and shapes by hand.
4. Push a straw, pen, or other thin object through ornament at top to make a hole for hanging.
5. Bake ornaments for one hour in oven at low setting.
6. Allow to cool.
7. Decorate. You can use markers, non-toxic acrylics or other type of paints, and glitter. Be creative.
8. Coat ornaments with a clear protective coating.
9. Put ornament hanger/ribbon through hole and hang.

Wreath: Mash cauliflower, instead of potatoes, and spread in a circle on plate. On top of the mash, arrange kale leaves to form a wreath. Decorate with fruits, nuts, seeds, and other veggies of your choosing. Then use dried tomatoes or cherry tomatoes to form a bow.

Mashed cauliflower

Kale leaves or spinach

Cherry tomatoes

Other fruits, veggies, nuts & seeds

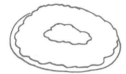
Spread mashed cauliflower on a plate

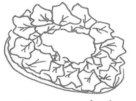
Arrange kale leaves on top.

Place on top the cherry tomatoes, seeds, nuts, and other fruits and veggies to decorate your wreath.

*You can use a round container or a bunt mold.

*Remember to ask an adult for help whenever you are cutting, slicing, or peeling.

Notes

Introduction

1. The American Heart Association, "Understanding Childhood Obesity: 2011 Statistical Sourcebook," 2011, 3.
2. The American Heart Association, "Overweight in Children," Getting Healthy, last updated November 7, 2013, http://www.heart.org/HEARTORG/GettingHealthy /HealthierKids/ChildhoodObesity/Overweight-in-Children_UCM_304054 _Article.jsp.
3. Centers for Disease Control, "Basics About Childhood Obesity," Overweight and Obesity: Childhood Overweight and Obesity, last updated April 27, 2012: http:// www.cdc.gov/obesity/childhood/basics.html.
4. Wasim Maziak, Kenneth Ward, and M. B. Stockton, "Childhood obesity: are we missing the big picture?" The International Association for the Study of Obesity, obesity review, 2007, http://www.scts-sy.org/files/documents/publications/Maziak ,%20obesity%20review_OBR.pdf.
5. Ibid.
6. The American Heart Association, "Overweight in Children."

Chapter 1

1. Traci Mann, et al., "Medicare's Search for Effective Obesity Treatments: Diets Are Not the Answer," *American Psychologist*, vol. 62, no. 3 (April 2007), 230–233, doi: 10.1037/0003-066X.62.3.220.

2. Stuart Wolpert, "Dieting Does Not Work, UCLA Researchers Report," UCLA Newsroom, news release, April 3, 2007, http://newsroom.ucla.edu/portal/ucla /dieting-does-not-work-ucla-researchers-7832.aspx.

3. John Naish, "Why Dieting Makes You FAT: Research shows trying to lose weight alters your brain and hormones so you're doomed to pile it on again," *Daily Mail*, April 23, 2012, http://www.dailymail.co.uk/health/article-2134162/Research -shows-trying-lose-weight-alters-brain-hormones-youre-doomed-pile-again.html.

4. Tom Valeo, "Does dieting make you fat?" *Tampa Bay Times*, April 24, 2012, http://www .tampabay.com/news/aging/lifetimes/does-dieting-make-you-fat/1226118.

5. Ibid.

6. William Anderson, "How Dieting Makes People Obese," *The Huffington Post*, August 13, 2012, http://www.huffingtonpost.com/william-anderson-ma-lmhc /weight -loss_b_1763559.html.

7. Ibid.

8. Melinda Johnson, "The Diet Mentality Paradox: Why Dieting Can Make You Fat," *US News & World Report*, August 17, 2012, http://health.usnews.com/health-news /blogs/eat-run/2012/08/17/the-diet-mentality-paradox-why-dieting-can-make -you-fat.

9. Ibid.

10. Ibid.

Chapter 2

1. Tara Parker-Pope, "The Fat Trap," *The New York Times*, December 28, 2011, http://www.nytimes.com/2012/01/01/magazine/tara-parker-pope-fat-trap.html ?pagewanted=all&_r=0.

2. Alexandria Sifferlin, "Study: Obese Kids Have Less Sensitive Taste Buds," Health & Family, *Time*, September 20, 2012, http://healthland.time.com/2012/09/20/study -obese-kids-have-less-sensitive-taste-buds/.

3. Rockefeller University, "Jeffrey Friedman, Discoverer of leptin, receives Gairdner, Passano awards," press release, April 13, 2005, http://newswire.rockefeller.edu/2005 /04/13/jeffrey-friedman-discoverer-of-leptin-receives-gairdner-passano-awards/.

4. WashingtonsBlog.com, "The real cause of the global obesity epidemic," March 17, 2012, http://www.washingtonsblog.com/2012/03/the-real-cause-of-the-global-obesity -epidemic.html; Nicholas D. Kristof, "How chemicals affect us," *The New York Times*, May 2, 2012, http://www.nytimes.com /2012/05/03/opinion/kristof-how -chemicals-change-us.html.

Chapter 3

1. Michael Moss, "The extraordinary science of addictive junk food" *The New York Times*, February 20, 2013, http://www.nytimes.com/2013/02/24/magazine/the -extraordinary-science-of-junk-food.html.

2. David S. Ludwig, Karen E. Peterson, Steven L. Gortmaker, "Relation between consumption of sugar-sweetened drinks and childhood obesity: a prospective, observational analysis," *The Lancet*, vol. 357, no. 9255 (February 2001), 505–508, doi: 10.1016/S0140-6736(00)04041-1.

3. Let's Move, "Learn the Facts," Partnership for a New America, accessed January 28, 2014, http://www.letsmove.gov/learn-facts/epidemic-childhood-obesity.

4. Face the Facts USA, "The sweet life and what it costs us," The George Washington University project, School of Media and Public Affairs, December 21, 2012, http:// www.facethefactsusa.org/facts/the-sweet-life-and-what-it-costs-us.

5. Isaac Eliaz, "Are you chronically dehydrated?" *Rodale News*, last updated August 7, 2012, http://www.rodale.com/chronic-dehydration.

6. Hopkins Children's, "Too Much Water Raises Seizure Risk in Babies," May 1, 2008, http://www.hopkinschildrens.org/newsdetail.aspx?id=4844.

7. Julie Armstrong and John J. Reilly, "Breastfeeding and lowering the risk of childhood obesity," *The Lancet*, vol. 359, no. 9322 (June 2002), 2003–2004, doi:10.1016/S0140 -6736(02)08837-2.

8. Eleanor Tidswell and S. Langley-Evans, "The health benefits of breastfeeding on the risk of children developing allergic asthma," *Journal of Human Nutrition and Dietetics*, vol. 24, no. 3 (2012), 307.

9. Lindsey Rennick Salone, William F. Vann, and Deborah L. Dee. "Breastfeeding: An overview of oral and general health benefits." *Journal of the American Dental Association*, vol. 144, no. 2 (February 1, 2013), 143–151, doi:10.14219/jada .archive.2013.0093.

10. Myles S. Faith, Barbara A. Dennison, Lynn S. Edmunds, and Howard H. Stratton, "Fruit Juice Intake Predicts Increased Adiposity Gain in Children from Low-Income Families: Weight Status-by-Environment Interaction," *Pediatrics*, vol. 118, no. 5 (November 1, 2006), 2066–2075, doi: 10.1542/peds.2006-1117.

11. Hamilton, Alissa, *Squeezed: What you don't know about orange juice* (Yale University Press, 2009).

12. Ibid.

13. David Heber, "Vegetables, fruits and phytoestrogens in the prevention of diseases," *Journal of Postgraduate Medicine* 2, vol. 50 (2004), 145–149.

14. Medline Plus, "Antioxidants," The U.S. National Library of Medicine, http://www .nlm.nih.gov/medlineplus/antioxidants.html.

15. Christine M. Williams, "Nutritional quality of organic food: shades of grey or shades of green?" *Proceedings of the Nutrition Society* 61, no. 1 (February 2002), 19–24: doi:10.1079/PNS2001126.

16. Environmental Working Group. "EWG's 2013 Shopper's Guide to Pesticides in Produce," http://www.ewg.org/foodnews/summary.php.

17. Edwin Simpser, "Feeding your child for lifelong health," *Journal of Pediatric Gastroenterology and Nutrition* 3, vol. 31 (2000), 329.

18. Susan B. Roberts and Melvin B. Heyman, *Feeding Your Child for Lifelong Health: Birth through Age Six* (New York: Random House Publishing Group, 1999).

19. Food Reference.com, "Children and Food Preferences," accessed February 12, 2014, http://www.foodreference.com/html/kids-food-preference-310.html.

20. Irene Chatoor, *When Your Child Won't Eat or Eats Too Much* (iUniverse, 2012).

21. Susie O'Brien, "Parents bribing kids into becoming fat," *Herald Sun*, June 1, 2012.

22. Leann L. Birch, "Development of food preferences," *Annual Review of Nutrition*, vol. 19 (July 1999), 41–62, doi: 10.1146/annurev.nutr.19.1.41.

23. Julie A. Mennella, Coren P. Jagnow, and Gary K. Beauchamp, "Prenatal and postnatal flavor learning by human infants," *Pediatrics*, vol. 107, no. 6 (June 1, 2001), e88 doi: 10.1542/peds.107.6.e88.

24. Dorothy Blair, "The Child in the Garden: An Evaluative Review of the Benefits of School Gardening," *The Journal of Environmental Education*, vol. 40, no. 2 (2009), doi: 10.3200/JOEE.40.2.15-38.

25. Michelle M. Ratcliffe, Kathleen A. Merrigan, Beatrice L. Rogers, and Jeanne P. Goldberg, "The Effects of School Garden Experiences on Middle School-Aged Students' Knowledge, Attitudes, and Behaviors Associated with Vegetable Consumption," *Health Promotion Practice*, vol. 12, no. 1 (October 21, 2009), 36–43, doi: 10.1177/1524839909349182.

26. Dina R. Rose, "Why Some Kids Should Play with Their Food," It's Not about Nutrition, August 30, 2011, http://itsnotaboutnutrition.squarespace.com/home /2011/8/30/why-some-kids-should-play-with-their-food.html.

27. Penny M. Kris-Etherton, William S. Harris, and Lawrence J. Appel, "Fish Consumption, Fish Oil, Omega-3 Fatty Acids, and Cardiovascular Disease," *Arteriosclerosis, Thrombosis, and Vascular Biology*, vol. 23, (2003), e20–e30, doi: 10.1161/01 .ATV.0000038493.65177.94.

28. Cynthia A. Daley, et al., "A review of fatty acid profiles and antioxidant content in grass-fed and grain-fed beef," *Nutritional Journal*, vol. 9, no. 10 (March 10, 2010), doi: 10.1186/1475-2891-9-10.

29. Renata Micha, Sarah K. Wallace, and Dariush Mozaffarian, "Red and Processed Meat Consumption and Risk of Incident Coronary Heart Disease, Stroke, and Diabetes Mellitus," *Circulation*, 121 (May 17, 2010), 2271–2283, doi: 10.1161/CIRCULA TIONAHA.109.924977.

30. Horace B. Powell, *The Original Has This Signature—W. K. Kellogg* (New Jersey: Prentice Hall, 1956).

31. K W Heaton, S N Marcus, P M Emmett, and C H Bolton, "Particle size of wheat, maize, and oat test meals: effects on plasma glucose and insulin responses and on the rate of starch digestion in vitro," *American Journal of Clinical Nutrition*, vol. 47, no. 4 (April 1988), 675–682.

32. K. L. Wrick, J. B. Robertson, P. J. Van Soest, B. A. Lewis, J. M. Rivers, D. A. Roe, and L. R. Hackler, "The Influence of Dietary Fiber Source on Human Intestinal Transit and Stool Output," *Journal of Nutrition*, vol. 113, no. 8 (1983), 1464–1479.

33. Erin E. Kershaw, Jeffrey and S. Flier, "Adipose Tissue as an Endocrine Organ," *The Journal of Clinical Endocrinology & Metabolism*, vol. 89, no. 6 (2004), 2548–2556, doi: 10.1210/jc.2004-0395.

34. Mayo Clinic Staff, "Omega-3 in fish: How eating fish helps your heart," The Mayo Clinic, 2010, http://www.mayoclinic.org/diseases-conditions/heart-disease/in-depth /omega-3/art-20045614.

35. Fred Ottoboni and Alice Ottoboni, "Can Attention Deficit-Hyperactivity Disorder Result from Nutritional Deficiency?" *Journal of American Physicians and Surgeons*, vol. 8, no. 2 (Summer 2003), http://www.jpands.org/vol8no2/ottoboni.pdf.

36. Greg M. Cole, Qlu-Lan Ma, and Sally A. Frautschy, "Dietary fatty acids and the aging brain," *Nutrition Reviews*, vol. 68, no. 2 (2010), 5102–5111.

37. Gina Kolata, "Gut Bacteria from Thin Humans Can Slim Mice Down," *The New York Times*, September 5, 2013, http://www.nytimes.com/2013/09/06/health/gut-bacteria-from-thin-humans-can-slim-mice-down.html.

38. Adam Marcus, "MSG linked to weight gain," Reuters Health, May 27, 2012, http://www.reuters.com/article/2011/05/27/us-msg-linked-weight-gain-idUSTRE 74Q5SJ20110527.

39. Debra Manzella, "Can Artificial Sweeteners Make You Gain Weight?" About.com, last updated February 20, 2008, http://diabetes.about.com/od/nutrition/qt/artifi cialsweet.htm.

40. Jon Gabriel, *The Gabriel Method*, (Beyond Words Publishing / Atria Books, 2007), 232.

Chapter 4

1. See Ellyn Satter's "Division of Responsibility in Feeding," EllynSatterInstitute.com; See also, Ellyn Satter "Your Child's Weight: Helping Without Harming." Wellness Councils for America's *Absolute Advantage* magazine, vol. 5, no. 6 (2006).

2. Sandra L. Hofferth and John F. Sandberg, "How American Children Spend Their Time," *Journal of Marriage and Family* 2, vol. 63, (May 2001), 295–308, doi: 10.1111 /j.1741-3737.2001.00295.x.

3. M. A. Cohn, and B. L. Fredrickson, "In search of durable positive psychology interventions: Predictors and consequences of long-term positive behavior change," *The Journal of Positive Psychology*, vol. 5, no. 5 (2010), 355–366: doi:10.1080/1743976 0.2010.508883.

4. Susie O'Brien, "Parents bribing kids into becoming fat," *Herald Sun*, June 1, 2012.

5. Amy T. Galloway, Laura M. Fiorito, Lori A. Francis, and Leann L. Birch, "Finish your soup: Counterproductive effects of pressuring children to eat on intake and affect," *Appetite*, vol. 46, no. 3 (May 2006), 318–323, doi: 10.1016/j.appet.2006 .01.019.

6. Amy E. Baughcum, Kathleen A. Burklow, Cindy M. Deeks, Scott W. Powers, and Robert C. Whitaker, "Maternal Feeding Practices and Childhood Obesity," *Archives of Pediatrics and Adolescent Medicine*, vol. 152, no. 10 (1998), 1010–1014, doi:10.1001/archpedi.152.10.1010.

Chapter 5

1. Sheldon Cohen and Denise Janicki-Devert, "Who's Stressed? Distributions of Psychological Stress in the United States in Probability Samples from 1983, 2006, and 2009," *Journal of Applied Social Psychology*, vol. 6, no. 42 (April 16, 2012), 1320–1334, doi: 10.1111/j.1559-1816.2012.00900.x.

2. Margot R. Solomon, "Eating as both coping and stressor in overweight control," *Journal of Advanced Nursing*, vol. 36, no. 4 (November 27, 2001), 563–573, doi: 10.1046/j.1365-2648.2001.02009.x.

3. Jay Kandiah, Melissa Yake, and Heather Willett, "Effects of Stress on Eating Practices Among Adults," *Family and Consumer Sciences Research Journal*, vol. 37, no. 1 (2008), 27–38, doi: 10.1177 /1077727X08322148.

4. Debra A. Zellner, Susan Loaiza, Zuleyma Gonzalez, Jaclyn Pita, Janira Morales, Deanna Pecora, and Amanda Wolf, "Food selection changes under stress," *Physical Behavior*, vol. 87, no. 4 (April 2006), 789–793, doi: 10.1016/j.physbeh.2006.01.014.

5. Jayne A. Fulkerson, Nancy E. Sherwood, Cheryl L. Perry, Dianne Neumark-Sztainer, and Mary Story, "Depressive symptoms and adolescent eating and health behaviors: A multifaceted view in a population-based sample," *Preventative Medicine*, vol. 38, no. 6 (2004), 865–875.

6. American Psychological Association, "Stress in America Findings," November 9, 2010.

7. Diana Bohmer, "Top 10 Sources of Stress for Kids," FamilyEducation.com, accessed February 12, 2014, http://life.familyeducation.com/stress/mental-health/36226.html.

8. Gianluca Gini and Tiziana Pozzoli, "Bullied Children and Psychosomatic Problems: A Meta-analysis," *Pediatrics*, vol. 132, no. 4 (October 2013), 720–29.

9. Simone Robers, Jijun Zhang, Jennifer Truman, and Thomas D. Synder, "Indicators of School Crime and Safety, 2011," National Center for Education Statistics, U.S. Department of Education, and Bureau of Justice Statistics, Office of Justice Programs, U.S. Department of Justice.

10. Medscape Education Diabetes & Endocrinology, "Bullying and obesity: An expert interview with Julie C. Lumeng," MedScape.org, released May 30, 2012, http://www.medscape.org/viewarticle/764371.

11. R. Reilly, "Bullying is bad for your health: Victims of playground taunts at SIX TIMES more likely to develop a serious illness in later life," Daily Mail, 2013, http://www.dailymail.co.uk/health/article -2397077/Bullying-bad-health-Victims -playground-taunts-times-likely-develop-illness-later-life.html

12. American Academy of Pediatrics, "Avoiding Bullying," HealthyChildren.org, 2013, http://www.healthychildren.org/English/safety-prevention/at-play/pages/Avoiding -Bullying.aspx.

13. American Academy of Pediatrics, "Helping children handle stress," 2013, http://www .healthychildren.org/English/healthy-living/emotional-wellness/pages/Helping -Children-Handle-Stress.aspx.

14. Brian Wansink and Ellen van Kleef, "Dinner rituals that correlate with child and adult BMI," *Obesity* (December 19, 2013), doi: 10.1002/oby.20629.

Chapter 6

1. National Council on Strength and Fitness, "Obesity and Inflammation," accessed February 12, 2014, http://www.ncsf.org/enew/articles/articles-obesityandinflammation.aspx.

2. Joseph Mercola and Rachael Droege, "How to Avoid the Ten Most Common Toxins," *Mercola Newsletter*, February 19, 2005.

3. Alice Park, "Exposure to Air Pollution in Pregnancy May Boost Chances of Obesity in Kids," *Time Health*, 2012, http://healthland.time.com/2012/04/17 /exposure-to-air-pollution-in-pregnancy-may-boost-chances-of-obese-kids.

4. U.S. Food and Drug Administration, "Update on Bisphenol A for Use in Food Contact Applications: January 2010," News Events, Public Health Focus, 2012, http://www.fda.gov/downloads/NewsEvents/PublicHealthFocus/UCM197778 .pdf.

5. Leonardo Trasande, Teresa M. Attina, Jan Blustein, "Association Between Urinary Bisphenol A Concentration and Obesity Prevalence in Children and Adolescents, *The Journal of the American Medical Association*, September 19, 2012, doi: 10.1001/2012.jama.11461; Alice Park, "BPA Linked with Obesity in Kids and Teens," *Time: Health & Family*, September 18, 2012, http://healthland.time.com /2012/09/18/bpa-linked-with-obesity-in-kids-and-teens/.

6. Joel Fuhrman, "Reverse Disease: Spotlight on Reversing and Preventing Disease," DrFurhman.com, accessed February 12, 2014, http://www.drfuhrman.com/disease /default.aspx.

7. Mike Adams, *Superfoods for Optimum Health: Chlorella and Spirulina* (Truth Publishing, 2009).

Chapter 7

1. Reite M, Ruddy J, and Nagel K, *Concise guide to evaluation and management of sleep disorders*, 3rd ed., (American Psychiatric Publishing, Inc., 2002).

2. National Sleep Foundation, *Sleep in America Bedroom Poll*, 2013, http://www.sleep-foundation.org/article/2013internationalbedroompoll.

3. Michael J. Breus, "Chronic Sleep Deprivation May Harm Health," WebMD.com, 2013, http://www.webmd.com/sleep-disorders/features/important-sleep-habits.

4. Avi Sadeh, Reut Gruber, Amiram Raviv, "The Effects of Sleep Restriction and Extension on School-Age Children: What a Difference an Hour Makes," *Child Development*, vol. 74, no. 2 (March 27, 2003), 444–455, doi:10.1111/1467-8624 .7402008.

5. Liz Neporent, "Childhood Obesity Linked to Lack of Sleep," January 23, 2011, http://abcnews.go.com/m/story?id=12743677.

6. Ibid.

7. Children's Anxiety Institute, "Sleep habits can affect levels of stress and anxiety in children and teens," ChildrenWithAnxiety.com, 2009, http://childrenwithanxiety .com/articles-resources/sleep-habits-can-affect-levels-of-stress-and-anxiety-in -children-and-teens.

8. Karen Spruyt and David Gozal, "A mediation model linking body weight, cognition, and sleep-disordered breathing," *American Journal of Respiratory and Critical Care Medicine* vol. 185, no. 2 (2012), 199–205, doi: 10.1164/rccm.201104-0721OC.

9. Kim Carollo, "Apnea Linked to Cognitive Problems," ABC News, November 3, 2011.

10. See "Sleep and Sleep Disorders," Centers for Disease Control and Prevention, last updated March 14, 2013, http://www.cdc.gov/sleep/.

11. Henry L. Shapiro, "Parenting Tips for Better Sleep," American Academy of Pediatrics, 2009, https://www2.aap.org/sections/dbpeds/pdf/sleeptips.pdf.

12. "Understanding OSA," Division of Sleep Medicine, Harvard Medical School, last reviewed November 8, 2010, http://healthysleep.med.harvard.edu/sleep-apnea /what-is-osa/understanding-osa.

13. Mayo Clinic Staff, "Diseases and Conditions: Obstructive sleep apnea," MayoClinic .org, June 15, 2013, http://www.mayoclinic.org/diseases-conditions/obstructive -sleep-apnea/basics/definition/con-20027941.

14. Eve Van Cauter and Kristen L. Knutson. "Sleep and the epidemic of obesity in children and adults." *European Journal of Endocrinology*, vol. 159, December 2008, doi: 10.1530/EJE-08-0298.

15. Carl E. Landhuis, Richie Poulton, David Welch, and Robert John Hancox, "Childhood Sleep Time and Long-Term Risk for Obesity: A 32-Year Prospective Birth Cohort Study." *Pediatrics*, vol. 122, no. 5 (November 1, 2008), 955–960, doi: 10.1542/peds.2007-3521.

16. Bill Hendrick, "Exercise Helps You Sleep: Regular Aerobic Exercise May Help Insomniacs," September 17, 2010, http://www.webmd.com/sleep-disorders/news/20100917 /exercise-helps-you-sleep.

17. Michael J. Breus, "Better sleep found by exercising on a regular basis," September 6, 2013, http://www.psychologytoday.com/blog/sleep-newzzz/201309/better-sleep -found-exercising-regular-basis-0.

Chapter 8

1. U.S. Department of Health and Human Services, *2008 Physical Activity Guidelines for Americans*, advisory committee report, http://www.health.gov/paguidelines/.

2. Karen H. Petty, Catherine L. Davis, Joseph Tkacz, Deborah Young-Hyman, and Jennifer L. Waller, "Exercise Effects on Depressive Symptoms and Self-Worth in Overweight Children: A Randomized Controlled Trial," *Journal of Pediatric Psychology*, vol. 34, no. 9 (October 2009), 929–939, doi: 10.1093/jpepsy/jsp007.

3. Eileen Eckeland, Frode Heian, Kare B. Hagen, Jo M. Abbott, and Lena Nordheim, "Exercise to improve self-esteem in children and young people," The Cochrane Library, January 26, 2004, doi: 10.1002/14651858.CD003683.pub2.

4. F.B. Ortega, J.R. Ruiz, M.J. Castillo, and M. Sjostrom, "Physical fitness in childhood and adolescence: a powerful marker of health," *International Journal of Obesity*, vol. 32, no. 1 (January 2008), 1–11, http://www.ncbi.nlm.nih.gov/pubmed /18043605.

5. Centers for Disease Control and Prevention, "How much physical activity do children need?" Physical Activity, CDC.gov, last updated November 9, 2011, http:// www.cdc.gov/physicalactivity/everyone/guidelines/children.html.

6. World Health Organization, "Global strategy on diet, physical activity, and health: Physical activity and young people," Information Sheets, 2014, http://www.who .int/dietphysicalactivity/factsheet _young_people/en/.

7. American Heart Association, "The AHA's Recommendations for Physical Activity in Children," Physical Activity and Children, updated January 17, 2014, http:// www.heart.org/HEARTORG/GettingHealthy/Physical-Activity-and-Children UCM_304053_Article.jsp.

8. Peggy J. Noonan, "Is your child getting enough physical activity?" *USA Today*, September 7, 2013, http://www.usatoday.com/story/news/health/2013/09/07/child -getting-enough-physical-activity/2777613/.

9. See CSIRO, "Kids Eat, Kids Play main survey begins," updated July 2012, http://www.csiro.au/Organisation-Structure/Divisions/Animal-Food-and-Health -Sciences/Health-wellbeing/Kids-Eat-Kids-Play-main-survey-begins.aspx.

10. Australian Institute of Family Studies, "The 2011 Longitudinal Study of Australian Children," annual statistical report, 2012, http://www.growingupinaustralia.gov .au/pubs/asr/2011/index.html.

11. Ibid. See also, American Heart Association, "Children's cardiovascular fitness declining worldwide: American Heart Association Meeting Report," abstract 13498 (room D163), November 19, 2013, http://newsroom.heart.org/news/childrens-cardio vascular-fitness-declining-worldwide.

12. Barbara A. Dennison, Theresa J. Russo, Patrick A. Burdick, and Paul L. Jenkins, "An Intervention to Reduce Television Viewing by Preschool Children," *JAMA Pediatrics (Archives of Pediatrics and Adolescent Medicine)*, vol. 158 (February 1, 2004) 170–176.

13. Tim Olds, Professor of Health Sciences, University of South Australia, quoted from the documentary Life at 7 (Heiress Films 2011), which partly documents the study *Growing Up in Australia: The Longitudinal Study of Australian Children*.

14. Amanda E. Staiano, Deirdre M. Harrington, Stephanie T. Broyles, Alok K. Gupta, and Peter T. Katzmarzyk. "Television, adiposity, and cardiometabolic risk in children and adolescents," *Preventative Medicine*, vol. 44, no. 1 (2013), 40–47, doi: 10.1016/j.amepre.2012.09.049.

15. Joseph Mercola, "Breakthrough Updates You Need To Know About Vitamin D," *Mercola Newsletter*, February 23, 2002.

16. Randy J. Seeley, Deborah L. Drazen, and Deborah J. Clegg, "The Critical Role of the Melanocortin System in the Control of Energy Balance," *Annual Review of Nutrition*, vol. 24 (July 2004), 133–149, doi: 10.1146/annurev.nutr.24.012003.132428.

17. X. Guillot, et al., "Vitamin D and inflammation," *Joint Bone Spine*, vol. 77, no. 6, (2010), 552–557.

18. Yong Zhang, Donald Y.M. Leung, Brittany N. Richers, Yusen Liu, Linda K. Remigio, David W. Riches, and Elena Goleva, "How Vitamin D inhibits inflammation," February 23, 2012, http://www.sciencedaily.com/releases/2012/02/120223103920.htm.

19. Christopher G.R. Perry, George J.F. Heigenhauser, Arend Bonen, and Lawrence L. Spriet, "High-intensity aerobic interval training increases fat and carbohydrate metabolic capacities in human skeletal muscle," *Applied Physiology, Nutrition, and Metabolism*, vol. 33, no. 6 (December 2008), 1112–1123, doi: 10.1139/H08-097.

20. Glenn A. Gaesser and Siddhartha S. Angadi, "High-intensity interval training for health and fitness: can less be more?" *Journal of Applied Physiology*, vol. 111, no. 6 (2011), 1540–1541, doi: 10.1152/japplphysiol.01237.2011.

21. Neil Neimark, "Five minute stress mastery," accessed February 14, 2014, http://www.thebodysoulconnection.com/EducationCenter/fight.html.

22. Izumi Tabata, et al., "Effects of moderate-intensity endurance and high-intensity intermittent training on anaerobic capacity and VO2max," *Medicine and Science in Sports and Exercise*, vol. 28, no. 10, (October 1996), 1327–1330.

23. Izumi Tabata, "Step By Step Guide on Tabata Training," May 1, 2011, http://tabatatraining.org/.

24. Neil Neimark, "Five minute stress mastery."

Chapter 9

1. Serpil Erermis, Nurcan Cetin, Muge Tamar, Nagehan Bukusoglu, Fisun Akdeniz, and Damla Goksen, "Is obesity a risk factor for psychopathology among adolescents?" *Pediatrics International*, vol. 46, no. 3 (May 18, 2004), 296–301, doi: 10.1111/j.1442-200x.2004.01882.

2. Lien Goossens, Caroline Braet, Leen Van Vlierberghe, and Saskia Mels, "Loss of control over eating in overweight youngsters: the role of anxiety, depression and emotional eating," *European Eating Disorders Review*, vol. 17, no. 1 (2009), 68–78, doi: 10.1002/erv.892.

3. Rhonda BeLue, Lori A. Francis, and Brendon Colaco, "Mental Health Problems and Overweight in a Nationally Representative Sample of Adolescents: Effects of Race and Ethnicity," *Pediatrics*, vol. 123, no. 2 (February 2009), 697–702, doi: 10.1542/peds.2008-0687.

4. Centers for Disease Control, Adverse Children Experiences (ACE) Study, www.cdc.gov/ace, last updated January 18, 2013.

5. Harvard Health Publications, "Understanding the stress response," Harvard Mental Health Letter, March 2011.

6. Robin Roberts, "The mind-body connection," Mind-Body Psychotherapy, accessed February 14, 2014, http://www.mindbodypsychotherapy.net/mbconnection.htm.

7. D.F. Williamson, et al., "Body weight and obesity in adults and self-reported abuse in childhood," *International Journal of Obesity*, vol. 26, no. 8, (August 2002), 1075–1082, doi: 10.1038/sj.ijo.0802038.

8. Barbara A. Dennison, Theresa J. Russo, Patrick A. Burdick, and Paul L. Jenkins, "An Intervention to Reduce Television Viewing by Preschool Children," *Archives of Pediatrics and Adolescent Medicine*, vol. 158, no. 2 (March 2004), 170–176, doi: 10.1001/archpedi.158.2.170.

9. Jeffrey G. Johnson, Patricia Cohen, Elizabeth M. Smailes, Stephanie Kasen, and Judith S. Brook, "Television viewing and aggressive behavior during adolescence and adulthood," *Science* 29, vol. 295, no. 5564 (March 2002), 2468–2471, doi: 10.1126/science.1062929.

10. Ibid.

11. Medscape Education Diabetes & Endocrinology, "Bullying and obesity: An expert interview with Julie C. Lumeng," MedScape.org, released May 30, 2012, http://www.medscape.org/viewarticle/764371.

Chapter 10

1. Jay Kandiah, Melissa Yake, and Heather Willett "Effects of Stress on Eating Practices Among Adults," *Family and Consumer Sciences Research Journal* 1, vol. 37(September 2008), 27–38, doi: 10.1177/1077727X08322148.

2. Debra A. Zellner, Susan Loaiza, Zuleyma Gonzalez, Jaclyn Pita, Janira Morales, Deanna Pecora, and Amanda Wolf, "Food Selection Changes Under Stress,"

Physical Behavior, vol. 87, no. 4 (April 2006), 789–793, doi: 10.1016/j.phys beh.2006.01.014.

3. Jayne A. Fulkerson, Nancy E. Sherwood, Cheryl L. Perry, Dianne Neumark-Sztainer, and Mary Story, "Depressive symptoms and adolescent eating and health behaviors: A multifaceted view in a population-based sample," *Preventative Medicine*, vol. 38, no. 6 (2004), 865–875, 10.1016/j.ypmed.2003.12.028.

4. Lisa M. Shin, Scott L. Rauch, and Roger K. Pitman, "Amygdala, Medial Prefrontal Cortex, and Hippocampal Function in PTSD," *Annals, New York Academy of Sciences*, vol. 1071, (July 2006), 67–79, doi: 10.1196/annals.1364.007.

5. Association for Psychological Science, "Understanding role of stress in just about everything," January 11, 2008, Science Daily, http://www.sciencedaily.com/releases/2008/01/080108152439.htm.

6. Tonya L. Jacobs, et al., "Self-Reported Mindfulness and Cortisol During a Shamatha Meditation Retreat," *Health Psychology*, vol. 32, no. 10 (March 25, 2013), 1104–1109, doi: 10.1037/a0031362.

7. Jeanne Dalen, Bruce W. Smith, Brian M. Shelley, Anita Lee Sloan, Lisa Leahigh, and Debbie Begay, "Pilot study: Mindful Eating and Living (MEAL)," *Complementary Therapies in Medicine*, vol. 18, no. 6 (2010), 260–264, doi: 10.1016/j.ctim.2010.09.008.

8. Karen L. Caldwell, Michael J. Baime, and Ruth Q. Wolever, "Mindfulness Based Approaches to Obesity and Weight Loss Maintenance," *Journal of Mental Health Counseling*, vol. 34, no. 3 (September 24, 2012), 269.

9. Claire Bates, "The World's Happiest Man," *Daily Mail*, October 31, 2012. http://www.dailymail.co.uk/health/article-2225634/Is-worlds-happiest-man-Brain-scans-reveal-French-monk-abnormally-large-capacity-joy-meditation.html.

10. Ibid.

11. Tonya L. Jacobs, et al., "Intensive meditation training, immune cell telomerase activity, and psychological mediators," *Psychoneuroendocrinology*, vol. 36, no. 5 (June 2011), 664–681, doi: 10.1016/j.psyneuen.2010.09.010.

12. The Mayo Clinic, "Meditation: A simple, fast way to reduce stress," 2011, http://www.mayoclinic.com/health/meditation/HQ01070.

13. Angie LeVan, "Seeing is believing: The power of visualization," *Psychology Today*, (December 2, 2009), http://www.psychologytoday.com/blog/flourish/200912/seeing-is-believing-the-power-visualization.

14. Steven Ungerleider and Jacqueline M. Golding, "Mental Practice among Olympic Athletes," *Perceptual and Motor Skills*, vol. 72, no. 3 (June 1991), 1007–1017, doi: 10.2466/pms.1991.72.3.1007.

15. Iris Martin, "Guided Visualization: A Way to Relax, Reduce Stress, and More!" PsychCentral, 2006, http://psychcentral.com/libguided-visualization-a-way-to-relax -reduce-stress -and-more/000684.

16. Joy A. Weydert, Daniel E. Shapiro, Sari A. Acra, Cynthia J. Monheim, Andrea S. Chambers, and Thomas M. Ball, "Evaluation of guided imagery as treatment for recurrent abdominal pain in children: A randomized controlled trial," *BMC Peditrics*, vol. 29, no. 6 (November 6, 2006), doi: 10.1186/1471-2431-6-29.

17. Miranda A.L. van Tilburg, et al., "Audio-recorded guided imagery treatment reduces functional abdominal pain in children: A pilot study," *Pediatrics*, vol. 124, (October 12, 2009) e890, doi: 10.1542/peds.2009-0028.

18. The Norwegian University of Science and Technology (NTNU), "Brain waves and meditation," *Science Daily*, March 31, 2010, http://www.sciencedaily.com/releases /2010/03/100319210631.htm.

19. Isabel L. Beck, McKeown, and G. McKeown, "Text talk: Capturing the benefits of read-aloud experiences for young children," *The Reading Teacher*, vol. 55, no. 1 (September 2001).

Chapter 11

1. Lisa A. Sutherland, et al., "Like Parent, Like Child," *Archives of Pediatrics and Adolescent Medicine*, vol. 162, no. 11 (2008), 1063–1069, doi: 10.1001/archpedi .162.11.1063.

2. Patrick Casey, et al., "Maternal Depression, Changing Public Assistance, Food Security, and Child Health Status," *Pediatrics*, vol. 113, no. 2, (2004), 298–304, doi: 10.1542/peds.113.2.298.

3. Stephen M. Petterson and Alison B. Albers, "Effects of poverty and maternal depression on early child development," *Child Development*, vol. 72, no. 6 (November/ December 2001), 1794–1813.

Chapter 12

1. Jemin Kim and Salomon Amar, "Periodontal disease and systemic conditions: a bidirectional relationship," *Odontology*, vol. 94, no. 1 (September 2006), 10–21, doi: 10.1007/s10266-006-0060-6.

2. Centers for Disease Control and Prevention, "Childhood obesity facts," Adolescent and School Health, last updated July 10, 2013, http://www.cdc.gov/healthyyouth /obesity/facts.htm.

Resource A:
Dr. Riba's Health Club

The mission of Dr. Riba's Health Club (DrRHC) is to promote healthy lifestyles in children, families, and communities by addressing medical, nutritional, social, economic, and behavioral issues in a comprehensive, compassionate, and empowering manner.

Founded in 2002 by Dr. Patricia A. Riba, Dr. Riba's Health Club (DrRHC) specializes in children of all ages, from newborns to eighteen-year-olds, and their families, taking a comprehensive approach to the prevention and treatment of childhood overweight, obesity, diabetes, and Failure to Thrive (FTT), a condition referring to children with delayed growth and development due to improper nutrition and an inability to maintain a healthy weight. DrRHC offers a variety of programs and services aimed at addressing the health needs of children and their families most at risk for obesity and diabetes. DrRHC reaches over 4,000 underserved families annually, targeting low-income areas in Orange County, California, where obesity and diabetes are serious concerns.

Dr. Patricia was honored as a 2010 "Agent of Change" by the Children and Families Commission of Orange County and received an "Excellence in Philanthropy Award" from the Orange County Community Foundation. Most recently, Dr. Patricia earned the CalOptima 2012 Circle of Care Award for excellence in quality service and Senator Lou Correa's Woman Making a Difference Award in 2013.

Program Descriptions

Health Club:

DrRHC approaches diagnosis, treatment, and prevention with a multidisciplinary team, providing direct patient care and individual treatment programs that are tailored to each child's needs. The multidisciplinary team is comprised of a pediatrician/medical director, registered dietitians, case manager, and fitness instructors. DrRHC treats the most severe cases of obesity and FTT.

DrRHC works to address the root causes of overweight and obesity, rather than just the symptoms, to ensure that the entire family is stronger and healthier. The overall intervention is the same for both overweight children and those with FTT:

1. Discuss the psychology of feeding
2. Teach families how to improve their nutrition
3. Promote increased physical activity
4. Assess and treat any medical or psychological comorbidities

With the nutrition counseling and fitness training provided by our multidisciplinary team at medical visits, our most recent evaluation in 2013 found that 84.5 percent of patients improved their body mass index (BMI) percentiles.

Fit Club™

Fit Club is an after-school and summer program serving low-income children ages four through eighteen and integrates physical activity, nutrition education, and healthy cooking classes/demonstrations. Afternoon sessions are available year-round.

The Fit Club summer program had amazing results. In 2010, 87 percent of children decreased their BMI, and improvements in fitness scores were statistically significant across all measures.

PC-Fit™

PC-Fit (Parent-Child Feeding Interaction Therapy) treats dysfunctional feeding-dynamic issues within families through live-coaching intervention in collaboration with the Child Guidance Center. This novel program is modeled after PCIT (Parent-Child Interaction Therapy), a live coaching intervention that strengthens the parent-child bond and provides highly consistent, appropriate, and effective parenting strategies. The rationale behind the strategies of PC-Fit is that children reflect their parents' attitudes and associations with food. The coach observes and coaches parent-child interactions over the course of multiple sessions during simulated family meal times through a one-way mirror while the parent wears a wireless earpiece. This program not only empowers parents to make mealtimes more enjoyable, but helps create a positive dynamic for the entire family to relieve tension at the dinner table with everyone enjoying meals together.

Fit Scouts™

In its newest program, Fit Scouts is a group of girls or boys who are dedicated to having a healthy heart through nutrition, exercise, and helping others. The program meets once a month and encourages young children to become active members in their community through various activities, field trips, exercises, and health lessons that correspond with that month's holiday, season, or theme. The troop is encouraged to carry out their core virtues throughout the month and can earn rewards to fill their "buckets" by doing various heart-healthy activities. This program is currently being piloted and will serve as a template to help girls or boys across the country to develop life-long healthy habits in a very fun way and bring those messages into their families.

Educational Programs

DrRHC encourages teaching obesity prevention and health concepts at an early age through specially designed classes on health and nutrition for parents of young children, with classes offered at preschools and other sites. Through a partnership with the Pretend City Children's Museum, DrRHC has designed fieldtrips for young children to learn about health and nutrition in a fun learning environment.

Medical Provider Education and Training

DrRHC believes that provider education and training make an important and necessary contribution to community health. Dr. Patricia conducts weight management training for providers at school districts and hospitals throughout the state. Provider education and training programs foster improved understanding of the psychology of and appropriate nutrition for feeding children, which is not generally discussed in medical school or residency programs.

To learn more about our programs and how you can help our team fight to prevent and treat obesity for families with scarce resources, or to start a Fit Scouts troop in your community, please go to our website www.DrRibasHealth Club.org.

Resource B:
Free Support Materials

Jon Gabriel & The Gabriel Method

Thank you for your interest in Fit Kids Revolution.

Both Dr. Riba and I are committed to helping you raise the healthiest, happiest kids in the world. The Gabriel Method is a leader in mind-body weight loss worldwide, and we offer dozens of educational and supporting resources that teach everything from healthy cooking to meditation.

To help support you in the process of raising healthy kids, I'd like to offer you two of my most popular resources.

- The first is access to three of my favorite recipes for kids, including photos and complete instructions.
- The second is for you (because your health is important too). It's my evening visualization practice, used by over 350,000 people nightly.

To access these bonuses, please visit: www.TheGabrielMethod.com/FitKids.

Thanks again for your interest and commitment to your family's health and wellbeing. I hope to connect with you online very soon.

In health,
—Jon Gabriel

Dr. Patricia Ronald Riba & Dr. Riba's Health Club

Thank you for your interest in Fit Kids Revolution.

Both Jon and I want to continue to support you as you try to implement strategies set forth in this book.

I'd like to share some additional resources for you and your family.

- The first is a set of printable placemats by season, which include: games, pictures to color, word searches, fun facts, and table talk questions. This is just another way to garnish fun at mealtimes to stimulate meaningful, pleasant conversations at the dinner table.
- The second bonus is access to a three-day meal plan with different food options, practical advice, and step-by-step instructions.

To access your bonuses, please visit: www.DrRibasHealthClub.org/FitKids.

Thanks again for taking the time to improve you and your family's health. I look forward to connecting with you online.

Warm wishes,
—Dr. Patricia Ronald Riba